T0260658

ANTHONY CERAMI

ANTHONY CERAMI

A Life in Translational Medicine

CONRAD KEATING

RUTGERS UNIVERSITY PRESS
New Brunswick, Camden, and Newark, New Jersey, and London

Library of Congress Cataloging-in-Publication Data
Names: Keating, Conrad, author.
Title: Anthony Cerami: a life in translational medicine / Conrad Keating.
Description: New Brunswick: Rutgers University Press, [2021] | Includes
    bibliographical references and index.
Identifiers: LCCN 2020051457 | ISBN 9781978801400 (cloth) | ISBN 9781978801424
    (epub) | ISBN 9781978801431 (mobi) | ISBN 9781978801448 (pdf)
Subjects: LCSH: Cerami, Anthony, 1940—Health. | Medicine—Research. |
    Biochemists—Biography. | Medical scientists—Biography. | Drug—Design.
Classification: LCC R850 .K43 2021 | DDC 610.72—dc23
LC record available at https://lccn.loc.gov/2020051457

A British Cataloging-in-Publication record for this book is available from the British
Library.

www.rutgersuniversitypress.org

Manufactured in the United States of America

To my wife, Jennifer

CONTENTS

CONTENTS

FOREWORD

I first met Professor Anthony Cerami forty years ago. It was in early December 1979, just a week or two before fall semester finals in my senior undergraduate year at Yale University. I had to come to New York to interview for the MD-PhD medical scientist training program, run jointly between Cornell and Rockefeller Universities, with a dream of becoming a graduate student (then called "biomedical fellows") there.

I was excited about my interviews. Beginning in the late 1970s and throughout the 1980s, The Rockefeller University had become the epicenter of the new science of molecular parasitology. Some of the world's most important and distinguished senior scientists on the Rockefeller campus were pioneering the applications of modern molecular biology to eukaryotic parasites. In the 1970s, William Trager and James Jensen had published in *Science* the continuous cultivation of human malaria parasites; Miklos Muller had discovered the hydrogenosome, a unique organelle found in *Tritrichomonas*; Nadia Nogueira and Zanvil Cohn worked out mechanisms for host recognition and destruction for the trypanosome causing Chagas disease; and Miki Rifkin found how human serum lysed the African trypanosomes causing cattle wasting. For me, there was really no other university or research institution that was as committed to cutting-edge science for the poor.

I was passionate about studying parasitic and tropical infections, and hoped to meld this interest with my Yale undergraduate major in molecular biophysics and biochemistry. This was an exciting time in science—the first genes had been cloned in the 1970s, and I aspired to apply this new molecular biology to the study of medically important parasites.[1] Not many scientists were interested in molecular parasitology, because parasites were mostly infectious agents affecting people living in extreme poverty, especially in the developing countries of Africa, Asia, and Latin America. The biotech revolution was just beginning, with Genentech becoming the first publicly traded biotech in 1980, but this new movement was largely focused on curing the diseases of North America, Europe, and Japan. There was an urgent need to apply biotech for diseases of the poor.

Of all the Rockefeller professors beginning to meld molecular biology with parasitology and tropical medicine, Tony Cerami was perhaps one of the most dynamic. I still remember meeting Tony Cerami for the first time during my MD-PhD interviews. At thirty-nine, he was probably the youngest full professor at The Rockefeller University and maybe one of the youngest Rockefeller full professors in its modern history. During my initial interview and later as a first-year student when we would meet regularly on Friday mornings, Tony was able to articulate a unique approach and vision for the biomedical sciences.

First and foremost, Tony is passionate about conquering illness. His approach, which he has successfully directed toward understanding everything from diabetes to aging, cystic fibrosis, tissue injury and repair, and even human African sleeping sickness, is to elucidate the fundamental biochemical flaws that allow an illness to take hold and then to design specific cures or preventions. As a young Rockefeller professor, he established what would become the renowned (and appropriately named) Laboratory of Medical Biochemistry (LMB). For me, what was unique about the LMB was that it was not beholden to specific technologies or even fields. Unlike most of the other Rockefeller laboratories that were focused around, say, immunology, genetics, or cell biology, Tony's LMB was truly interdisciplinary. It was located initially in the basement of Theobald Smith Hall, one of the founding laboratories of the Rockefeller Institute of Medical Research built in the early 1900s, but later LMB relocated to the then new tower building in the Rockefeller campus. There, working day and night, were a group of scientists, each with widely divergent talents. They included organic chemists, immunologists, molecular biologists, pathologists, and even some biochemists. The idea was that scientists of diverse backgrounds worked together to solve fundamental problems in disease mechanisms. Through this approach, Tony and his protégés were seldom restricted to specific fields of research. Instead, it was recognized that conquering disease was the goal, and this required a truly interdisciplinary approach.

While at Rockefeller, Tony became one of the first principal investigators and lab heads with a laser focus on translational medicine and well before the term had actually come into fashion. After meeting Tony that December day, I remembered how we were soon finishing each other's sentences, and I had my life's calling—to take the LMB approach toward solving parasitic and tropical infections, also now sometimes referred to as neglected tropical diseases, or NTDs. Today, I also try to instill in my laboratory scientists the importance of focusing on a disease and designing unique and specific vaccine targets. We now have vaccines for human hookworm infection and schistosomiasis in clinical trials, as well as at least a half dozen other diseases, ranging from Chagas disease and leishmaniasis to Middle East respiratory syndrome and Severe acute respiratory syndrome coronavirus infection, which will hopefully enter the clinic soon.

In retrospect, I was one of many of Tony's former students, postdoctoral fellows, and senior scientists who became committed experts in translational medicine, with each of us pursuing our own diseases or groups of diseases. Today, there is an impressive list of scientists who have spent formative years in Tony's LMB or later, after Tony left The Rockefeller University to establish the Picower Institute of Medical Research. Included among the stars on the list are Nina Schor, the current deputy director of the National Institute of Neurologic Disorders and Stroke (NINDS) of the U.S. National Institutes of Health (NIH); the Nobel Laureate Bruce Beutler; and major professors (in no particular order) at Yale University (Richard Bucala), Washington University St. Louis (Daniel Goldberg), University of Dundee (Alan Fairlamb), University of North Carolina (Steven Meshnick),

Jichi Medical University (Masanobu Kawakami), University of Michigan (Ronald Koenig), Feinstein Institute (Kevin Tracey), Columbia University (Joseph Graziano), Albert Einstein College of Medicine (Michael Brownlee), Boston Children's Hospital (Christina Luedke), and many others!

Beyond the laboratory, Tony Cerami also taught me how science can become an important force for social change. He was a close personal friend of the late Kenneth S. Warren, who, in his leadership role at the Rockefeller Foundation, established a network of scientists to promote the field of tropical infectious diseases. Tony was a founding scientist in this new Rockefeller Foundation initiative, and he was instrumental in elevating the entire field of neglected diseases. This bigger approach introduced me to strong role models for embarking on important initiatives that extended beyond my laboratory. They inspired me to pursue initiatives such as providing access to essential medicines for neglected diseases still affecting hundreds of millions of people, uncovering a previously hidden burden of poverty-related diseases in poor areas of the southern United States, and now fighting a well-organized and funded antivaccine lobby in America.

In this sense, I have always felt that scientific bravery represented one of Tony's greatest attributes, and something that he passed on to the next generation of his mentees. He seldom walked away from tackling an important problem due to limitations in his current expertise or the talents of his scientific staff. Instead, Tony displayed scientific bravery by introducing new technologies or approaches for the expressed purpose of promoting translational medicine and solving disease problems. In so doing, he generated paradigm shifts for a variety of key disease targets, and in many respects, he helped to lay the foundation of modern translational medicine. It has been an honor for me to have Anthony Cerami as my thesis adviser, mentor, and valuable colleague and friend!

Peter Hotez, MD, PhD
Professor of Pediatrics and Molecular Virology, Texas Children's Hospital,
Endowed Chair in Tropical Pediatrics, and Dean, National School
of Tropical Medicine, Baylor College of Medicine

ANTHONY CERAMI

INTRODUCTION

In 1978, on a hot airless afternoon, while lying defeated and prostrate in a manure-splattered corral in Kenya, the American biochemist Anthony Cerami experienced a scientific epiphany. The brief "Eureka" moment, which would subsequently be regarded as critical in bringing about a revolution in therapeutics, came as the direct result of an embarrassing and catastrophic failure. As a proponent of "rational drug design," Cerami had traveled from his laboratory at The Rockefeller University, New York, to East Africa convinced that he had found an effective treatment for a wasting disease in cows caused by parasites. However, after many successful experiments under laboratory conditions, when he eventually administered the drug to infected animals in the wild, instead of providing the expected cure, it in fact caused the animals' rapid demise.

At the most intense moment of discouragement, while sitting in the corral engulfed by a sense of failure, Cerami slowly began to piece together elements of the disastrous therapeutic experiment in an attempt to make biological sense of what had happened. Why, he asked himself, would nature allow the wasting away of animals to occur? And how could parasites cause the wasting and death of European cows, whereas African antelopes with a similar parasitic load did not develop a degenerative illness and die? Then suddenly and unannounced came a flash of insight, hitting Cerami "like a brick."[1] The cow was killing itself as the direct result of an inappropriate immune reaction to the presence of foreign organisms. The parasite was not the problem. The real issue, Cerami reasoned, was that the body was making something that caused the animal to waste away. For more than a century, as a direct response to the insights of the immunologist and Nobel laureate Elie Metchnikoff, it had been understood that the immune system could recognize molecules that were foreign to the body—"nonself" in the language of immunology—and mount an attack on the invader. In reaction to the therapeutic failure in the corral, Cerami made an observation of perhaps equal biological significance: he hypothesized that this mediator could be an endogenous cause of human disease; under certain circumstances, the body was capable of attacking itself.

As a scientist, Cerami was a systems thinker, someone who excelled at pattern recognition, and, with the malodorous stench of cow manure still lingering in his nostrils, over the course of the next thirty minutes, he sketched the outline of a scientific plan that over the coming decades would have a profound effect on the health of millions of patients across the world who suffer from chronic inflammatory diseases. Returning to his Laboratory of Medical Biochemistry, Cerami set himself and his colleagues a critical question: what was this mediator, and how could its action be prevented? Within a decade, the laboratory had identified the mediator as a protein that we know today as tumor necrosis factor (TNF), an inflammatory molecule that plays an important role in a number of human diseases, including shock, rheumatoid arthritis, and Crohn's disease. Crucially, the scientific team also reasoned that if the protein could be neutralized, they could potentially treat any number of infectious, chronic and immunological diseases.

The corral in Kenya proved to be a frontier between parasitology and immunology, reflective of the fact that innumerous scientific discoveries are made at the intersections of two or more disciplines. In the bigger scheme, it also became not only a crucial location in the development of Cerami's career but also a site of immense importance in the development of a whole new branch of medicine. Fifty years ago, Cerami was a pioneer, an outlier for a new approach in biomedical science; although not medically qualified, he was deeply interested in finding new therapies for previously unmet medical need. The scientific process of bringing disease-targeted knowledge from the laboratory to treat patients in the clinic became known as "translation" or "translational medicine" and emerged at a time when the science of drug discovery was undergoing a profound methodological change. The rapid application of technologies developed in medical genetics and molecular biology had led to a corresponding recalibration in thinking and scientific direction: long-established routes of discovering chemical drugs unpredictably by the empirical method of trial and error had begun to be undermined, even "tainted," by their "very simplicity"[2] and displaced by a more targeted, rational approach, with the use of monoclonal antibodies in the form of injectable "biologic" therapeutics. As we shall see in the following chapters, the Eureka moment that occurred in East Africa not only catalyzed new areas of translational research but also resonated within the world of biotechnology, was deeply interconnected with the development of molecular biology, and provided the conceptual breakthrough that contributed to anti-TNF therapy becoming the world's best-selling pharmaceutical drug class, with sales in excess of $26 billion per year.[3]

Few would have thought when Cerami was born in rural New Jersey in 1940 that his career would intersect so consequentially with the rise of translational medicine. Interested in the mechanisms of disease from an early age on his parents' chicken farm, he went on to study biochemistry at The Rockefeller University before beginning to work in more detail on treatments for diabetes, blood disorders (including sickle cell disease), the biochemistry of aging, the wasting disease cachexia, and the biology of accelerating nerve regeneration, in each case attempting to link discoveries in the laboratory to the eventual development of physical treatments for patients in a clinical setting. Quite why this was so novel and groundbreaking becomes apparent only by looking more closely at what the existing state of drug discovery was when Cerami began work, at a moment when established techniques began to fall under question.

One of the earliest references to translational research can be found in the title of an article by Karp and McCaffrey in 1994, reporting on a meeting of the National Cancer Institute workshop that examined ways to improve the clinical outcomes for leukemias and lymphomas. "Any impact on curability and duration and quality of survival will be achieved only by building on the cumulative knowledge accrued at multiple levels—molecular and cellular levels as well as in the intact patient— and augmenting the momentum of the bidirectional exchange of information between the laboratory and the clinic that has characterized leukemia research from its incipience."[4] For Karp and McCaffrey, translational research, with its emphasis on a "bidirectional" concept of so-called bench-to-bedside factors, rep- resented a new approach to patient care and one that flew in the face of older laboratory-based practices that treated drug discovery as an abstract endeavor or something that was the outcome of trial-and-error empiricism. The difference in approaches spoke to an intriguing conundrum at the heart of twentieth-century drug discovery and of medical science in general: what is the most effective driver of scientific advance? What modes of activity generate the steps forward in the understanding and treatment of diseases that modern societies have come to rely on? While translating biological knowledge from the workbench to the bedside has always in some respects been an essential part of the practice of medicine, in the pretranslation era, the answer had largely been weighted toward "basic" sci- ence: curiosity-based endeavors not necessarily directed at a particular clinical endpoint, based almost exclusively in a laboratory rather than clinical setting, and usually resulting in the creation of sets of abstract theories, patterns, and ideas. In the words of Gerald Edelman, winner of the Nobel Prize in 1972 for his work on antibodies, "basic research is a kind of hunt for a general principle that underlies a whole set of phenomena, and since the universe doesn't seem to be constructed the way a library is constructed, you don't always know exactly what you're look- ing for."[5] Basic science is something of a game of chance, given its unpredictability. Such work, the production of principles and knowledge, is nevertheless the bed- rock upon which the discipline develops. The alternative perspective, and the one that had caught Karp and McCaffrey's attention, was translational science: a form of applied research that set out with the express objective of tackling a specific medical problem and that sought to unite abstract, theoretical science with practi- cal application, very often practiced by "physician-scientists" who understood enough about scientific exploration to apply its technology at the bedside.[6] This was, in other words, the process of translating theory into practice: targeting spe- cific diseases from the outset and seeking practical outcomes in the form of treat- ments to be used at the bedside on real patients.

While the terminology to describe this new type of research only came into being in the 1990s, the shift to disease-centered translation was already in evidence by the time that a young Cerami came to work with Kenneth S. Warren, the evangelical parasitologist and director of health sciences at the Rockefeller Foundation in the 1970s. In 1978, Warren launched the influential Great Neglected Diseases of Mankind Program (GND), which sought to introduce modern biomedical science (molecular and cell biology, genetics, and immunology) to the study of infectious diseases in low-income countries. In his quest to bring the most cost-effective health care to the world's poorest people, Warren recruited to the GND leading biomedical scientists, including the molecular geneticist David Weatherall, the immunologist John David, the immunochemist Emanuela Handman, and Anthony Cerami. Many had never worked in the field of parasitology before, but they were all determined to use medical science to help address the disproportionate inequity of the global poor. Importantly, the program affirmed one of Warren's ideals, that a significant part of the investigators' efforts would be spent in applied collaborative research with colleagues in low-income countries. In this sense, the project would establish global networks linking "the bench to the bush"[7] and lay the foundations for a model of medicine in low-income countries at both basic and applied levels. Crucially, the "bench to the bush" model was a prototype of the integrated approach favored in translational medicine that was beginning to be practiced by large universities and institutes around the globe. Fueling the new discipline was a widespread belief at the time that the momentum of the bidirectional exchange of information between the laboratory and the clinic had slowed and that the application of the new discipline of translational medicine was required to accelerate the translation of biomedical discoveries for the better prevention, diagnosis, and treatment of diseases.

The rise of translational medicine also owed much not only to dissatisfactions with previous methods of drug discovery in basic science but also to the new availability of technologies, most notably the application of the new sciences of molecular and cell biology to study human diseases. The new discipline of molecular biology had developed rapidly in the 1950s and 1960s, beginning to reveal how genetic information is passed from generation to generation and how individual cells function, both as self-contained units and as parts of the intricate communications network that forms the basis of life itself.[8] Although major scientific achievements do not always have immediate practical benefits, there was a growing recognition by the 1970s that molecular biology had the potential to catapult the medical sciences into an exciting and more productive era. Gradually, a shift of emphasis was discernible, from the study of disease at the level of patients or their diseased organs to the study of their cells and molecules.[9] In turn, this opened new possibilities for research—the ability, for instance, to target specific human diseases at a molecular level, which further reinforced the move away from abstract, haphazard, trial-and-error drug discovery toward rational drug design. For his part, Cerami recognized that if he was going to understand mechanisms of disease and the chemical basis of aging at the molecular and cellular level, he needed to be able to isolate, purify, and determine the structure and function of the basic molecules of life—the proteins of which we are formed and the enzymes and mediators that drive the chemical reactions responsible for the normal function of our organs. In this sense, Cerami was very much a biomedical researcher shaped by the mores of his day and the scientific culture emerging at the bench of the Rockefeller laboratories as defined by the teachings of Peyton Rous, Maclyn McCarty, George Palade, Robert Bruce Merrifield, and Detlev Bronk. His training reached deep into basic science, yet, drawing on this expertise, he established himself at the forefront of the new field, regarded as the quintessential translational scientist, who defined the pathogenesis of disease in the laboratory and used that knowledge to discover treatments for patients at the bedside.

By the turn of the new millennium, the shifts that had been under way in drug discovery for several decades, with Cerami at the forefront, were recognized at international and institutional levels. Translation had gone mainstream, becoming *the* accepted and indeed preferred method of biomedical research. In the words of the clinical epidemiologist Stephen H. Woolf, in a perceptive article in the *Journal of the American Medical Association*, 2008, "translational research means different things to different people, but it seems important to almost everyone."[10] Woolf went on to describe just how significant translation was to the scientific community in light of the decision by the National Institutes of Health (NIH) to make translational research a priority by launching the Clinical and Translational Science Award (CTSA) in 2006. As the largest biomedical research institution in the world, the NIH, by championing a translational approach aligned to a major new source of funding, ultimately shaped the research programs of hospitals, research institutes, universities, and concentrated the minds of biomedical scientists across the United States and beyond.

Nor was the NIH the only national science institute to embrace the translational pathway. In 2007, Colin Blakemore, the chief executive of the British Medical Research Council (MRC), argued for an all-out commitment to clinical research and to the translation of basic science into benefits for patients. The infrastructure, designed to accelerate the findings of pure research into medical advances, was to be provided by the founding of six new MRC translational medicine centers, geographically spread across the United Kingdom.[11] The six centers would focus on different areas of medical research: epidemiology, neuromuscular diseases, global health, obesity, transplantation, and disease surveillance. In addition, Blakemore announced that the MRC planned to invent, develop, and market its own drugs—with or without industry support—to speed up advances against rare diseases and those that mainly affected developing countries.

The move by the NIH and MRC to embrace translation was indicative of growing anxieties at the beginning of the twenty-first century that the advances being made in the laboratory, particularly in the fields of molecular medicine and genetics, were not resulting in the expected new wave of drugs to treat the seemingly intractable—and often common—diseases of our modern lifestyles: including heart disease, cancers, and strokes. Some of the difficulties here lay in the field of translation itself and required not only the renewed financial support of major international research institutions but also a degree of careful introspection within translational research about the methods and models being used. The growing sense of relative stagnation and the desire to hasten innovation was not confined to the NIH and MRC: it was also felt within the corridors of the pharmaceutical industry. In 2007, Chas Bountra was head of biology at GlaxoSmithKline (GSK), where he led a group of 230 highly motivated scientists working across gastro-intestinal, inflammatory, and neuropsychiatric diseases, with the aim of discovering therapeutic drugs. "You know," Bountra reflected, "at GSK we only really started talking about translational medicine around the year 2000. And the reason was about that time, more and more of us in the industry realized that the sorts of things that we do in the lab—cellular assays, and studies in animal models—when we took them into Phase 1 and Phase 2 studies they didn't work! What became apparent was that there was a gap in translation."[12] Bountra set about identifying the main factors responsible for this bench-to-bedside translational failure. First, he came to believe that very high-quality molecules that had given positive results in animal models and cellular assays in the lab failed because they were adminis-tered to the wrong set of patients. He reasoned that most diseases are diverse in character. For example, Alzheimer's is not a single disease and has amorphous symp-toms; in 100 patients, some might be depressed, some are agitated, and others will not be able to recognize their children. Similarly, multiple sclerosis is not a single disease; there are numerous subsets, and essentially patients are very heteroge-neous. There are not only factors such as age, sex, weight, and ethnicity to con-sider; there is also a genetic element at play in many diseases (even with respect to viral diseases such as COVID-19). Second, Bountra believed that a longstanding problem was that when molecules were taken into the clinic, they were often administered at the wrong dose. With an animal model in the laboratory, it is a relatively easy procedure to ramp up the dose until there is a response. In the clinic, patients might complain about the side effects of nausea or neuropathy, whereas it is difficult to pick up these reactions in a rat or a mouse. Third, Bountra felt that translation was hampered because the biomarkers used to identify or evaluate the presence of a disease in the clinic were often not sensitive enough, especially in relation to neurological diseases such as depression. Appointed to the chair of translational medicine at the University of Oxford in 2008, Bountra's experience of working in both the pharmaceutical industry and in academic medicine led him to some clear conclusions: "I think most animal models are a waste of time. I do not think that getting efficacy in a six inch furry animal with a six inch tail is going to predict what will happen in a large heterogeneous group [of humans]. For me, translational medicine is about how do we get greater confidence that what we find out in the lab will actually translate into patients in the clinic?"[13]

A transformative step in gaining that confidence and avoiding knowledge being lost in translation came when an international consortium that included the NIH and The Wellcome Trust completed the Human Genome Project (HGP) in 2003.

The $3 billion undertaking has been one of the major biological revolutions of the modern era; through its sequencing of DNA, the HGP has made possible the investigation of bodies, genetics, and diseases on a scale hitherto unimagined, rooted in a mapping of all the genes of the human genome.[14] This has been an invaluable aid not only to understanding diseases but also to designing medications and the more accurate prediction of their effects. Most important, the project represented the latest step in the type of precision medicine that lies at the heart of translational research: of the specific targeting of particular diseases at a molecular level.

Into the dynamic and rapidly evolving world of translational medicine, this book sets the life of Anthony Cerami. Cerami's story and that of the evolution of translation are intimately entwined: the contours of Cerami's career shaped by developments in translation and, in exchange, the field itself molded by Cerami's work. To understand one is to understand the other. By examining the life of this often overlooked biochemist, it is possible to intimately focus on the ideas and thought processes of a scientist who has helped to define the great acceleration in translational research over the past fifty years—research that, knowingly or otherwise, has most likely affected the life of almost everyone on the planet. We also gain a better understanding of the febrile creative atmosphere that percolated through the laboratories leading the way in translational science, as well as gain insight into the art, science, successes, failures, and providence that underlie major scientific breakthroughs. Anybody interested in the questions of where modern medicines come from, how health outcomes around the globe are affected by research and imagination, and where the future of drug discovery and biologics is leading will be rewarded by exploring Cerami's life in translation.

At its most basic, Cerami's life story—however esoteric the science of biochemistry might seem at the outset—is a highly recognizable journey through human endeavor: moments of optimism balanced by forces of discouragement, creativity, and disillusionment; the excitement of discovery tempered by long periods of unrewarded labor. The equilibrium of this scientific career was kept in check partially by Cerami's breadth of interests and his willingness to engage in new areas of research beyond his initial expertise. The focus of his attentions shifted dramatically and, at times, rapidly: from parasitology to genetic disease, from antibodies to aging, from common ailments to orphan diseases. He saw no fundamental reason why he as a scientist could not learn to prevent sickle cell disease, the complications arising from diabetes, parasitic affliction, disease processes, and even human aging. The aim was to move beyond observations of the natural world in order to perform experiments that would produce new diagnostics and therapeutics. While some might see in this a degree of intellectual flightiness, this was rather a type of self-preservation: the flexibility necessary to build a lengthy and productive career. Although his name is probably most synonymous with the discovery of TNF, a molecule responsible for several destructive aspects of chronic inflammation (and subsequent work to inhibit this molecule in humans), and which went on to make Cerami's reputation and forge a multibillion dollar industry in the therapeutic treatment of rheumatoid arthritis, one of his greatest attributes as a biomedical scientist has in fact been this diversity of interest and his cultivation of a cross-disciplinary approach to biomedical investigation. Cerami believed that a research team is more confident of success if it is able to approach problems from a variety of perspectives and scales. As one of his colleagues, Masanobu Kawakami, has written, "I was [also] surprised to see so many projects were ongoing in so many different disciplines. It took me years to understand that they were all related in his mind and that his interest was focused on entire systems instead of single organs or traditional isolated disciplines."[15] This scientific attitude was reflected in the composition of various iterations of his "laboratory-without-walls," first at The Rockefeller University, the Picower Institute, and later Warren Pharmaceuticals and Araim Pharmaceuticals. Each lab included investigators with expertise in chemistry, biology, and medicine, all of whom were guided by the doctrine that the broader the thought process, the better, given that one never knew in advance where insights were going to come from. This leitmotif was echoed by Sir Aaron Klug, the Nobel laureate and leader of the Laboratory of Molecular Biology in Cambridge (United Kingdom). Klug advised young scientists to "equip yourself to do a wider range of things than you are actually interested in immediately. You never know what might pay off."[16]

Making use of in-depth interviews with Cerami himself alongside unprecedented access to his personal archive, as well as a series of conversations with a whole cohort of clinicians, basic scientists, discovery scientists, lawyers, supporters, and detractors based around the world, and conducted between 2013 and 2020, this volume offers the first in-depth exploration of Cerami's life in translational medicine. As with any biographical work, this is by necessity a partial view; it aims not to document every moment of Cerami's life but rather to apply a spotlight to the development of his career and the parallel growth of the field to which he contributed so much. In doing so, we also of course uncover the human stories behind the science. Reflecting Cerami's interests, the range of material under consideration here is considerable, from molecular biology, human health, and the rise of biotechnology to philanthropy, scrupulous and unscrupulous business practices, and the protective power of the legal system. Moreover, just as translational medicine encompasses and connects multiple constituencies—academics, physicians, patients, pharmaceutical companies—so Cerami's life spans similar groups. He himself chose to make his career at the intersection of academic science, business, and biotechnology: he was an entrepreneur, realistic about pursuing science in the age of capitalism. In many ways, he saw money as a way of pursuing science, and he was uninhibited about working with venture capitalists, creating spin-off companies, or establishing scientific institutes. This worked both ways: translational research is expensive; it has a limitless appetite for financial support. Likewise, the economic rewards that could be generated by the development of successful treatments were potentially immense. Beyond the science, then, exploring Cerami's life brings into focus some of the critical issues in modern discovery: How to raise capital for risky projects? How to protect intellectual property? Should medical treatments developed for the benefit of humanity be patented? And how to create the most conducive atmosphere for ideas to flourish? By uncovering the new, the unknown, and the unexpected, Cerami's life in translation continues to influence the present day and beyond.

1 · HARD WORK

Anthony Cerami was born on October 3, 1940, in Newark, New Jersey. He spent his childhood, in what was then the rural isolation of his parents' small chicken farm, near the town of Pine Brook. Both his parents were first-generation U.S. citizens, whose lives were testament to social and cultural forces that brought about the great wave of European migration in the preceding century. His parents' families lived in the township of Nutley, New Jersey, which had been settled by the Dutch and English, starting in the late 1600s. In the middle of the nineteenth century, Irish and Italian immigrants arrived to work in the local quarries that supplied brownstone to major cities like New York, as well as the mills in New Jersey. Into this bustle of human industry and whirling cacophony of community, Tony spent the first eight years of his life.

Both his paternal grandparents were born in Sicily, and his father, Anthony—who had a middle name but no one knew exactly what it was—was born in 1910, in Nutley. His mother, Hazel Kirk, was born in 1914, of English and Irish parents, reflecting the cosmopolitan makeup of Nutley's immigrant diaspora. Neither of Tony's parents had education beyond the third grade: both could read and write and do simple arithmetic; however, they occupied a position in society that necessitated their early entrance into the workforce. This economic imperative did not dilute their determination to secure better schooling for their children, for they knew implicitly the value of a good education without ever having had the opportunity to have one themselves.

Just as the United States had been demographically shaped by the push-and-pull factors affecting Europe, New Jersey in the postwar period reflected national population trends. According to the U.S. Census, in 1920, 50 percent of all Americans lived in urban areas, and between 1940 and 1950, the population increased by 14.5 percent to over 150 million. Between 1950 and 1980, there was a flight from the densely populated city centers to suburban neighborhoods and a general trend westward. This direction of travel was not only followed but also taken one geographical step further by the Cerami family, and in 1948, Cerami the boy left the bustle of Nutley life for the bucolic setting of Fine Soil farm (eponymously renamed "Judy Lynn Farm" after the birth of his sister).

In part, Cerami's life is the quintessence of the American Dream. Born into self-confessed "humble" circumstances, through a combination of natural ability, luck, and determination, he went on to become a member of the nation's scientific elite when, in 1972, he was appointed head of the Laboratory of Medical Biochemistry at The Rockefeller University. In science, or indeed in any field of endeavor, the timeline of an individual's interest in the subject that will dominate their lives often begins in childhood. Historians have found it difficult to productively liberate the contribution and experiences of children in the past, but understanding the historical world of the extraordinariness of *ordinary* life might begin by appreciating that the axis of most people's worlds was the family. This was certainly the case for the boy "Tony," and his early life gives expression to what one historian terms "the voice of the unheard"[1] by describing, in the historical moment, past patterns of experience and the material conditions of life that are now a vanished part of time and place.

For not only was Tony a much-loved child, but his labor was indispensable to the survival of the family farm, and it is a story that conforms to a wider tapestry of agricultural life in the United States during the first half of the twentieth century. As he recalled, "My parents needed me to work just to keep the farm going, without me they couldn't have done it. And in terms of the food that we ate, we raised all of it ourselves. There were chickens, pigs, turkeys and ducks so we did quite well; we weren't starving or anything."[2] By 1951, living standards for many Americans were rising, due in part to the preeminence of the United States in the postwar world, and it was also the same year that Tony's sister, Judith, was born. Economics is an important factor in determining fertility rates: during the boom years, between 1946 and 1964, the birth rate doubled for third children and tripled for fourth children, although this national trend was not played out in the Cerami household, and Judith was the only addition to the Cerami family. Nonetheless, Judith's arrival brought with it an added economic cost. The financial burden of rearing and educating farm children[3] was a study undertaken by agricultural historian James Tarver to accurately reflect, at prices prevailing in 1954, the true costs of *birth, food, clothing, education,* and *labor contribution of children* in the United States. It was not merely some cold-blooded exercise in actuarial science; it framed the cadence and realities for families in pursuit of happiness in rural America.

O. E. Baker made the first published study of the costs of rearing farm children.[4] He estimated that it cost $2,500 during 1922–30 to rear and educate the average child on farms in the United States to the age of fifteen. By allowing $50 per year for the labor contribution from ten to fifteen years of age, the cost of rearing and educating children was reduced by $250, to a net expense of $2,000. Twenty-seven years later, Tarver found that "the average annual value of a boy's labor, age 14 and 15, in 1954 was $325."[5] The boy, Tony, was fourteen in 1954, and this aggregate sum seems less than his overall contribution to the family economy. One of his jobs seemed particularly onerous: "I would sit for 12 hours in a darkened room candling

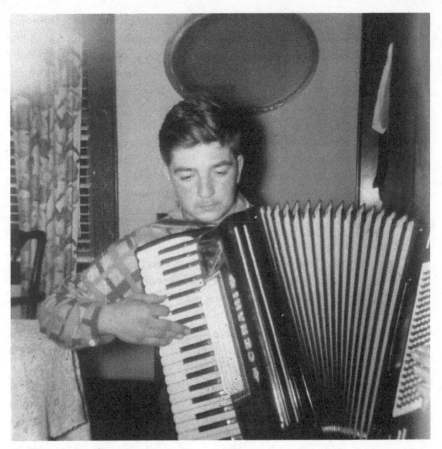

Cerami with accordion. Circa 1949.

eggs, picking out the cracked, or old eggs or those with blood spots, only the best eggs were sent to the market or you could be penalized." The values and attributes that later defined Cerami's scientific attitude were being forged in the crucible of monotonous and oppressive farm work. The Stakhanovite energy, the sheer horsepower he had for hard labor, and the belief in the necessity of perseverance would all serve him well during those inevitable intense moments of discouragement and years of hard, lonely work associated with science.[6]

Admittedly, there were vacillations in early life as Tony sought to find his place in the world. The secret gyroscopes in his mind were affected by two destabilizing forces: early exposure to rudimentary rural education and an inner confusion as to his own identity. One of Tony's first efforts at systematic observation took place in Pine Brook Grammar School, where eight grades were taught in four rooms with little regard to education, except the preparation of students for unskilled work. Studious by nature, the child sought intellectual stimulation outside the stultifying classroom, and salvation came in the form of the traveling county library, which had been converted from a former bread truck. By chance, one of the books that the child happened to select was *The Autobiography of Benjamin Franklin*. This book inspired him to dream that although he came from an undeniably modest background, he might live an original life of creativity and discovery. Tellingly, sixty years later, reflecting back on his early life in rural New Jersey, he wrote, "This book has given me the courage to escape from the bondage of financial and intellectual poverty."[7] In a different light, but no less fundamental in the development of his character, Cerami's early life was dominated by a sense that he never truly fitted in, and by his own admission, "I didn't know who I was." This feeling of being conflicted may be partly explained by his mother's insistence on bringing him up as a Protestant because she felt Catholicism was antiquated, yet the Italian diaspora in which he moved was overwhelmingly Catholic. Moreover, he was conscious that having an Italian surname—even though he was half English—made him overly self-conscious at a time when discrimination against Italian Americans was rife and institutionalized. He stood on the threshold of a new challenge.

The psychotherapist Sigmund Freud recognized that the self-belief necessary to set out a chosen path can be created in an individual by the intervention of a respected, significant figure. Freud termed this altruistic act as the placing of "a golden seed," noting that at some stage in their formative years, most successful people remember someone telling them that they possessed an exceptional talent. For Tony, that formative person was his teacher Mr. Arthur B. White, at Caldwell High School, New Jersey. Attending school in the town of Caldwell involved a daily 40-mile roundtrip for Tony from his home in Pine Brook, but the two hours that he spent every day in Mr. White's agriculture and science classes were to prove life-altering. Arthur White was not a big man, but he was tough, fair, and unconsciously exuded a quiet authority that all the high school students respected. And it was not just the studiously natured young Tony that Mr. White helped; he dedicated himself with just as much enthusiasm to encouraging less gifted students. Perhaps having himself lived through the economic privations of the Great Depression in 1930s Illinois, he understood better than most the arduous monotony of work on a family farm. Mr. White taught vocational agriculture, and he encouraged Tony's studies in mathematics, algebra, trigonometry, and, most important, biology. Tony excelled academically, and his sense of self and his place in the world began to crystallize during the four years he spent at Caldwell High School. His fate was sealed, as he began to sense the scale of his own talent. Arthur White took his responsibilities seriously, and he was committed to all students who enjoyed science, but he was also a mentor in other important ways. From White, Tony learned "respect for people who were on the margins; he was free of prejudice, and he imparted that to me. I spent a quarter of my entire time at school in his classes, and it changed me; he was a good person, he saw something in me, and encouraged me to embark upon a scientific career."

One of the genuinely intriguing elements about life is that, yes, some people can identify an individual who had a profound influence on the course of their lives,

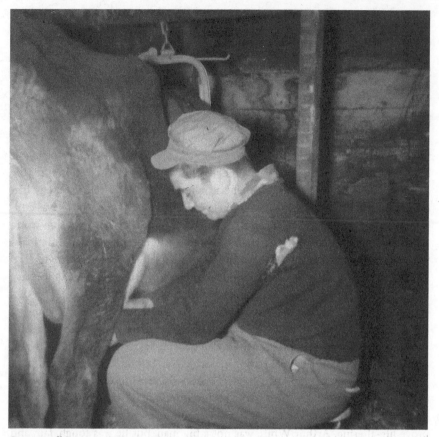

Cerami milking cow. Circa 1956.

but equally true is that no one can know in advance who these life-changing characters are going to be. These are completely unpredictable, stochastic encounters, only explicable by what statisticians term the "play of chance." Without the placing of the metaphorical golden seed by the inspirational Mr. White, it is probably true that Tony Cerami would not have made his life in science.

An intrinsic component of the vocational agriculture course at Caldwell High School was the organization Future Farmers of America (FFA). Established in the 1920s, the FFA sought to resuscitate a reconnection to rural life at a time when the younger generation was losing interest and leaving farming. One of the FFA's founders, Walter Newman, had a great vision, offering farm boys the opportunity for self-expression and the development of leadership skills in order to develop confidence in their own ability. With his feet firmly planted in rural life, the ideas incubating in Tony's mind immediately attracted him to the FFA. Their emphasis on conservation, animal husbandry, and improving agricultural methods struck a chord with the world he inhabited.

His rise within the FFA was prodigious, becoming the vice president for the state of New Jersey in 1957, and his attendance at the organization's annual meeting in Kansas City marked not only the first occasion the teenager had flown in an airplane but also the first time he had left his home state. Tony found the FFA socially ecumenical and free of any class or race discrimination. Its liberating ethos helped increase his understanding of biology and land conservation: it forged a lifelong belief in the altruistic rectitude of wanting to help people.

The FFA was the arena in which the teenager gained confidence in the art of public speaking, whether it was at the annual meeting in Kansas City or at state meetings when talking to local gatherings about agriculture's role in improving community life. Not content with the constraints of moral force persuasion, his consummate knowledge of animal husbandry brought him wide acclaim at agricultural fairs throughout New Jersey, where he happily judged and awarded prizes to outstanding milking cows, bulbous Thanksgiving turkeys, pigs, chickens, and riparian ducks.

It appeared that there were not enough hours in the day as Tony found the time to join another youth organization, the 4-H Club.[8] Set up at the beginning of the twentieth century to teach school children about science, leadership, and community service, the emphasis on personal growth and preparation for lifelong learning made it immediately attractive to the aspirational, far-sighted teenager. The humanitarian ideal of helping people and being in the service of others was given vivid direction from reading another book collected from the traveling book repository. The aim of the author was true and expertly targeted the young student's burgeoning scientific imagination. The book was Paul de Kruif's *Microbe Hunters*, a landmark in the history of science that presented, in effervescent prose, the stories of the first discoveries of disease agents, ways of transmission, and effective drugs for treatment. Because of Paul de Kruif's proselytizing zeal for science and clear descriptions of the significance of new scientific findings, hundreds of medical doctors, including several Nobel Prize winners, have described how reading this book helped them decide to study biomedical sciences.[9] Tony undeniably "got a lot out of the book," and it fired his imagination to think of the world, *his world*, as being thickly populated by living microbes, invisible to the human eye. The book presented Cerami's inquisitive mind with a scientific critique that he used to interrogate his own environment: what, for example, caused coccidiosis among the farm's chickens, which led to them wasting away and dying, and why did so many relatives on his mother's side of the family suffer and die of diabetes? Surely these would be as worthy targets for eradication as Texas fever or syphilis?

Many academically gifted children were born in rural United States in 1940, but few would go on to become members of the National Academy of Sciences, the nation's oldest scientific body. This is understandable, because all of us are shaped by our economic and cultural environment, and it is almost impossible to transcend these frontiers, some might say *barriers*, of our own expectations of life's possibilities or, indeed, the social settings that we inhabit. The working families of 1920s

Nutley did not expect to become international business executives or that their progeny would occupy positions of power within the governing political elite. Anthony Cerami senior, born in 1910, did not envisage a career as an architect, museum curator, or volcanologist; these possibilities could not be seen or imagined, and therefore they did not exist. They were beyond his grasp, outside of his line of vision—unknown, unachievable.

Compared to his father, Tony's life illustrates the accidental nature of human lives. For in Mr. White he had a patron, who, by encouraging ever higher academic standards, enabled Tony to stand on the threshold of a previously undreamed of possibility—a college education. Tony knew that his parents could not afford to pay college fees, but by securing a full scholarship, he was, in effect, paid to go to university. There would be other people who subsequently influenced Tony Cerami's life in science: Ed Reich, Irv Goldberg, and Ken Warren, among them, but without Mr. White, no science; without science, no Rockefeller career, no Rockefeller career, no life in translational medicine.

The universe and Cerami's place within it were expanding, and naturally, he studied agriculture, chemistry, and biochemistry at Rutgers University, the State University of New Jersey. He was the first person on both sides of his family to attend and graduate from university;[10] this was the springboard that allowed him to break free of social constraints, to accelerate the speed of upward mobility and to be the author of his own scientific journey. His arrival in science may have been accidental, but he was now gripped by the excitement of discovery, and he was determined to relentlessly continue to break new ground.

For the Irish poet Paul Muldoon, the terrain of his childhood, which he remembered as a beautiful part of the world, is returned to over and over again in his poetry, although he had not been back there for thirty years. Indeed, so deeply affected was he by this corner of Northern Ireland that he said it was "still the place that's burned into the retina." Possibly, many of us are held captive by our own past; likewise, there are an infinite variety of delusions by which we survive its inescapable reach, but what was certainly true is that Cerami's memory of farm life was at odds with the idyllic nostalgic inferences depicted in the work of the American artist Norman Rockwell. In the intervening years, between the rural childhood that shaped Cerami's worldview and occupying a position of power in biomedical science, he became a very wealthy man. This material well-being did not in any way dilute his efforts to use science to try to reduce the burden of disease, but the memory of those years when work was oppressive and money was in short supply may have gone deep in his psyche. This is certainly the belief of Mike Brines, Tony's long-term friend and scientific collaborator who feels that Cerami's connection to affluence is nuanced and not straightforward. "Honestly, I don't think money has made him happy. Happy to pursue some science, maybe. . . . He said he didn't want money, that it was a way of doing things. But I do think he is undermining the [influences] underlying his childhood, I think he's got a streak that is economical, on the one hand he spends money freely, but if he thinks that something is not a bargain, it bothers him. So I think that life on the farm has some remnant." Notwithstanding one's character and personality, no individual can remain immune from the vicissitudes of life. Some of these indiscriminate influences are conceived internally, products of nature, while others are exogenous in origin, determined by luck, chance, and environment. All of these variables played a significant role in shaping the intonation and direction of Cerami's life in translational medicine.

In some respects, Cerami's field of inquiry, the breadth of his interests, and his scientific evangelism resonate with the values and careers of two of his nineteenth-century heroes: Paul Ehrlich and Louis Pasteur. Both men—and Cerami—were realistic about pursuing science in the age of capitalism. They worked across a wide spectrum of interests and diseases; Ehrlich focused on antimicrobial chemotherapy, immunology, and hematology, while Pasteur absorbed himself in solving problems in the silk industry, the mining industry, vaccination, and rabies. One hundred years later, Cerami occupied a similar position at the frontiers of business and biology; he saw money as a way of pursuing science, and he was uninhibited about working with venture capitalists, creating spin-off companies, or establishing scientific institutes. He was an entrepreneur who sought to get discoveries made in the clinic to be translated, as safely and efficiently as possible, into drugs that could be used by patients in the clinic. The skill of hard work, and it is a skill, was learnt in childhood, as were other values that were immutable and whose influence proved impossible to escape.

2 · THE ROCKEFELLER EFFECT

I have zeal and ability, I am naturally talented—I am ambitious to become a
distinguished investigator.

—Elie Metchnikoff (in P. de Kruif, *Microbe Hunters*)

When in the fall of 1958, Cerami traveled to New Brunswick to study at
Rutgers University, he became part of a great social experiment that had its origins
in the colonial era. Founded in 1766, Rutgers University was subsequently granted
land-grant status in 1864. The establishment of land-grant colleges was in response
to the need to increase agricultural productivity by focusing on the teaching of
science, agrarian practices, and plant and soil improvement. Cerami's distinctive
scientific attitude had yet to solidify, but, as he later recalled, there was a real sym-
biosis between the institution's academic specialisms and his own innate interests.
"Naturally, because of my background, I studied agriculture at Rutgers University,
the State University of New Jersey"—an undertaking that was only made possible
through the acquisition of a full scholarship for the entire four years of the course.[1]

The scholarship, which covered essential living costs, needed to be augmented,
and Cerami worked assiduously throughout his undergraduate career. Twice a
week, he worked four-hour shifts as a college librarian, enabling him to earn money
and, more important, keep up with the scientific literature. At the same time, during the long summer vacations, the impecunious Cerami found a well-paid job
isolating anticancer drugs with the organist chemist, Dr. K. V. Rao, at Pfizer Pharmaceuticals in Maywood, New Jersey. The cancer research laboratories of Pfizer
were under the direction of John L. Davenport and operated in conjunction with
the National Cancer Institute to develop drugs to treat some forms of cancer. As
early as the 1920s, Pfizer chemists had learned of a fungus that fermented sugar to
citric acid and had gone on to commercialize the chemical production of citric
acid: subsequently, their expertise in fermentation technology was to prove critical in the mass production of penicillin in the 1940s.

The young Cerami began working at Pfizer in his sophomore year. The pay was
good and the overtime rates high, so he happily worked twelve- and fifteen-hour
days in the knowledge that he could make enough money in the summer vacation
to live for the rest of the year. The research at Pfizer, developing new forms of
chemotherapy for patients with cancer, was driven by the empirical method: the

methodical screening of many thousands of compounds until something was found that could target cancer cells. This pharmacological screening of disease states in animal models had been pioneered by Paul Ehrlich at the beginning of the twentieth century in his search for a "silver bullet" that targeted the microbes that cause syphilis but did not damage anything else in the patient's body. Working with the thoughtful, quiet, and diligent Dr. Rao, Cerami sought to isolate agents from fungal and bacterial products, including streptonigrin, but none registered positively on the therapeutic index, and most proved poisonous. This empirical approach led Cerami to conduct elixir-seeking experiments on some curious natural products: "one time we got a big shipment of large Osage oranges, they're green and have pulp inside and it was my job to chop them up and extract what I could. We found toxins but I don't think anything ever happened."[2] This was hands-on natural product chemistry, and the attempts to isolate potential anticancer therapeutics often involved Cerami running twenty-foot-tall chromatic vacuum columns to extract the fungal fermentation product that ran down the column. As many applied biomedical researchers will testify, drug discovery is not an exact science, and Pfizer's attempts to seek a panacea for cancer in natural product chemistry ultimately proved unsuccessful. The unpredictable empirical method did find compounds that killed cancer cells in a tumor, but they also killed the animal.

There are formative events that can be hidden by our subconscious, and the failure of the empirical screening techniques deployed by the Pfizer chemists may have been one experience that went onto shape Cerami's scientific modus operandi. Of course, he recognized that the role of luck and chance is often pivotal in medical innovation—the classic example being Alexander Fleming's discovery of a mysterious mold on a Petri dish that eventually led to the therapeutic discovery of penicillin by scientists in Oxford or William Campbell's use of fermentation techniques and the empirical screening of several thousand soil samples leading to a Nobel Prize and the discovery of ivermectin, a broad-spectrum antiparasitic drug.[3] While the Pfizer vacation job provided an early encounter with the inescapable play of luck and chance in science, if Cerami was to harness his desire to help people who were sick and truly embrace the excitement of discovery, a more scientifically predictable path would need to be found.

The British molecular biologist John Cairns has written that much of the pleasure of becoming a scientist comes from being part of a communal effort and being able to observe at close quarters the continual evolution in our understanding of the world around us.[4] It was this sense of being a privileged witness to a communal effort that became Cerami's source of greatest pleasure, something that was initially fostered both at university during term time and at the private lab during the summer. While the efforts to find effective cancer drugs for use in the clinic were unsuccessful, the scientific and social interactions made by Cerami in the Pfizer lab were instructive. The multinational workforce, composed in part of eastern European refugees from Latvia and Lithuania, offered him a new worldview of realpolitik that was novel and disarming. People talked in an unemotional, almost matter-of-fact way about the turbulent years of World War II, displacement, eternal exile, and the salvation and humanity that they often found in the world of science. These serendipitous encounters with such a diverse group of people at Pfizer made a deep impression: "I learned a lot there—it was an important part of my education although it wasn't part of my course work, and I learned [plenty] from the practical aspects of life and chemistry and, more importantly, how to work in a laboratory."[5]

Another early scientific influence on the young undergraduate was the chemist and entomologist Andrew Forgash, one of Cerami's many teachers at Rutgers. Forgash spent his entire academic career at the university, and as well as making a major contribution to the invention of the insect repellent DEET, he was an authority on how to prevent and control the outbreak of insect-borne diseases such as malaria, dengue fever, and trypanosomiasis, the disease caused by protozoan trypanosomes spread by the tsetse fly. Several decades later in the 1980s, the quest to identify new drugs to kill trypanosomes would provide Cerami with the opportunity to follow in the chemotherapeutic tradition of his scientific hero, Paul Ehrlich, which would ultimately define a new field of scientific inquiry and change clinical practice.

Beyond the work of Forgash, much inspiring and groundbreaking research was taking place at Rutgers in the early 1960s. The nutritional biochemist Hans Fisher advocated the idea that nutrition could be used to heal—or even prevent—disease. His fascination with amino acids set him on a path that placed him at the forefront of linking nutrition to health. Originally appointed by Rutgers Poultry Science department in 1954, he showed that knowledge of diseases of chickens provided an excellent model for studying disease in humans. Fisher advocated the benefits of a high-fiber diet as a defense against atherosclerosis, and Cerami was later to dedicate years of laboratory research to elucidating the theory that the nonenzymatic reaction of glucose with other body proteins was responsible for the complications of diabetes and some aspects of aging in general.[6] At Rutgers, for the first time, Cerami recognized that he had the ability to make connections across disciplines and to marry observation and imagination, just as those around him did. The invisible threads linking his scientific interests together began to catalyze.

But first, life had to be lived. The reality of day-to-day living at the all-male university—Rutgers became coed in 1970—suited Cerami, as his *hardscrabble* background had prepared him well for rudimentary dormitory living. At Rutgers, his housing was free, and fifteen students from the Agriculture School had shared bedrooms, a kitchen, and a dining room in the attic of a large old brownstone building. Childhood history, however, did not map exactly onto the experience of early adulthood at Rutgers. The political atmosphere was now far different from that in rural New Jersey: the easygoing nature of the early 1960s that heralded the start of a freer and more generous existence marked a poignant counterpoint to the murmurings of opposition to the Vietnam War that came to national prominence in 1965. Cerami was not immune to these countervailing currents, and in 1960, he joined the Reserve Officer Training Corp (ROTC) while still at Rutgers. After his two years' service, he did so well on the American history test that he was offered the rank of second lieutenant if he was willing to stay on. He declined the offer. The idea of the ROTC originated in the Morrill Act of 1862, which had established land-grant colleges. Part of the federal government's requirements for these institutions was that they included military history and strategy as part of their curriculum, forming what became known as the ROTC. Until the 1960s, many universities required compulsory ROTC for all of their male students. However, because of the protests against the Vietnam War, compulsion was dropped in favor of volunteer programs. Cerami was never overtly party political: he was far too immersed in science to engage in overt political activity, and any effort beyond his work was dedicated to a more pressing engagement. In early June 1962, Tony married his high school sweetheart, Katherine Lois Lindner, in Glen Ridge, New Jersey. Katherine taught science at a junior high school before changing her career to become a medical librarian.

The newly married Cerami was now twenty-two years old, about to graduate from Rutgers, and determined to forge a career in science. One sultry afternoon while sitting in hushed concentration in the local library, surrounded by open stacks filled with learned scientific journals, he picked up the prospectus of The Rockefeller Institute for Medical Research (RIMR). For over half a century, the RIMR had helped to shape the agenda for biomedical research and had become the foremost scientific location for highly educated, highly imaginative seekers of change.[7] After reading that the aim of the institution was the pursuit of unfettered scientific research, Cerami experienced what Darwin H. Stapleton describes as the "Rockefeller Effect,"[8] deciding on the spot that "this is where I would really like to go."[9]

In the early years of the twentieth century, the RIMR, under the influence of the American physician, scientist, and administrator Simon Flexner, had sought to bring workers and teachers from every part of the world into close and stimulating contact.[10] By the middle decades of the century, the Rockefeller Institute was seen as the nation's leading research organization in biomedical science, while its alumni were ubiquitous in the highest echelons of U.S. academic science. The distinctiveness of the RIMR was sustained by the inimitable leadership of the scientist, educator, and administrator Detlev Wulf Bronk, who became president in 1953. Bronk was a direct descendant of Jonas Bronck, the seventeenth-century Dutch trader, after whom the New York borough of the Bronx is named. Detlev Bronk was a scientist who became a visionary innovator in his chosen discipline of biophysics and combined this interest with his later careers as college president and scientific leader. In addition to being head of the National Academy of Sciences from 1950 to 1962, Dr. Bronk was president of the American Association for the Advancement of Science in 1952. He was also an adviser to Presidents Truman, Eisenhower, and Kennedy.[11] According to J. Rogers Hollingsworth in his excellent study of

Bronk's presidency at The Rockefeller University, "Bronk was a dreamer, a person whose ambitions for The University were virtually without limit."[12] Bronk built on the Institute's successes and then set it on a new path: in the future, it would not only be a center for research excellence but also provide graduate education for future scientific leaders of the nation. Because it would be a new type of training institution, the Rockefeller would retain its distinctive atmosphere. It was this combination of research and postgraduate excellence that would frame the next stage of Cerami's early career.

In 1953, when Bronk became president, the Institute structurally metamorphosed into a graduate university (the RIMR became The Rockefeller University in 1965) with the authority to grant the degrees of philosophy and doctor of medical science. Under Bronk's presidency from 1953 to 1968, the interdisciplinary approach was pushed to the fore, with the aim of producing scientists who had broad knowledge in a variety of fields and who were the antithesis of the "society split into the titular two cultures—namely the sciences and the humanities" described by C. P. Snow in 1959.[13] In 1961, Bronk outlined to the powerful Board of Trustees the type of educational environment he wanted to establish at York Avenue and 66th Street, suggesting that "it is unwholesome, and indeed dangerous for the future welfare of mankind, for scientists to live and work, to study and teach, in an environment in which they are not in close contact with creative, critical scholars in the humanities and arts. Such associations are a valuable quality of a university. Lack of such contact with those who help determine the future of civilization makes specialized research institutes barren intellectual environments."[14] While the university was too small to offer programs in the humanities, this could be offset by offering each student a generous stipend to be used to engage with the rich artistic life of New York City. Moreover, Bronk arranged for humanists and social scientists to present public lectures at the university and for music concerts to be held in its facilities.[15] Bronk's personal warmth and charisma were tangible to all those who met him, and this evoked strong feelings of loyalty and devotion to him and to the values that he espoused, especially among the cadre of graduates he selected to study at his beloved center of learning. In addition to his love of knowledge and of the necessity of creating the right environment where creative thinking can flourish, he was also a strong believer in the work ethic as championed by Eleanor Roosevelt, who once opined that "it is not more vacation we need—it is more vocation."

Another distinctive feature of the academic life that Cerami was about to enter at The Rockefeller University was the inverse ratio of graduate students to faculty, a phenomenon that had been accelerating under Bronk's presidency. By the early 1960s, there were about 100 graduate students and 400 members of faculty, and Bronk firmly believed that the selection of the student body should be every bit as rigorous as that of their professors. Accordingly, during his tenure, Bronk personally interviewed nearly all of the students before they were admitted. As Hollingsworth suggests, "The only students selected for admission were those whose commitment to advanced study and research was believed to be equal to that of the faculty. All students were considered to be intellectually mature, highly motivated, and capable of self-study."[16]

Sitting in the public library assiduously reading the prospectus of the RIMR, Cerami knew little about the intellectual stature and charisma of Detlev Bronk. All he knew was that if he wanted to study for a PhD in biochemistry, he had to write to the president. The RIMR admitted twenty-four students a year to the graduate program who had secured either an outstanding bachelor's or MD degree. Almost immediately, Cerami received a letter from Bronk inviting him for an interview, which would be held on the fourteen-acre campus, perched high in bustling Manhattan above the East River, with panoramic views of the borough of Queens. Simon Flexner had intended both the architecture and the principles of the institution to impress workers and teachers alike, and this was certainly the effect felt by the visiting Cerami: "Walking up the hill from the main gate at 66th Street and York Avenue you're struck by the imposing buildings. When I walked into the main building, Dr. Bronk was in a gigantic office. I was greeted by his executive secretary, Mabel Bright, who was very nice to me, and she sat me down. I waited for him to finish his phone conversation."[17] Despite the potentially overbearing surroundings, Cerami "really liked him, he was a wonderful man and treated me as an equal—he had a big effect on me."[18]

Before leaving the building, Cerami was told by Mabel Bright that the program's intake was capped at twenty-four students and that his application was in all probability too late. By his own admission, he proceeded to "lay it on pretty thick," recognizing intrinsically that Mabel Bright wielded a good deal of power. Every few days he would phone, reinforcing his presence in her mind. Following a week of telephonic persuasion, Cerami was accepted to become the twenty-fifth student in a class of twenty-four.[19] This marked a watershed moment in his development as a translational scientist: "It was Mabel Bright who convinced Dr. Bronk to accept an additional student, and that extra step she took made a tremendous difference to my life."[20] Bright's kindness was to mark the beginning of an enduring relationship, and when the opportunity arose to repay her generous intervention, Cerami was quick to act. When, after suffering a stroke, Detlev Bronk died in New York Hospital on November 17, 1975, Bright found herself in a precarious situation.[21] While the new president wanted to work with his own staff, The Rockefeller University was unwilling to retain her, and she had not yet reached retirement age. By this time, Cerami was already a young member of faculty at The Rockefeller University with his own laboratory, and when he realized that Bright was being forced to resign, he immediately hired her to oversee the day-to-day management of his lab, where management skills, honed over many years, made her a valuable member of his team for the next decade. Indeed, so great was his admiration for Mable Bright that when he became dean of graduate and postgraduate studies, he arranged for her to be presented with an honorary PhD. As he recalled, "you can imagine the kind of shit that I took when I told people what we were going to do. They said 'but she doesn't even have a bachelor's degree....' I didn't care: Mabel Bright was the core of the place, and she did more for the university than most of the people who were there. She was the heart of the program and a lot of people agreed with me. That was the story of Mabel Bright; she was an incredible person and one of the main people responsible for the graduate program at The Rockefeller University."[22]

Back in the summer of 1962, Cerami had his admittance to postgraduate study in hand and was preparing to join the powerhouse of American biomedical science. As an idealist, wanting to use his chosen field of biochemistry to help change the world, and from the outset nurturing a passion "to understand human diseases and explore new ways to treat them," he was perfectly matched to his new surroundings.[23] The Rockefeller University was a Mecca, a place that called the scientific faithful from across the globe and one that aimed to prepare young people to be scientific leaders of the nation. But what was to be Cerami's way forward: what would be his distinctive approach? The answer would take many years to fully materialize, yet already in 1962, Cerami was instinctively a systems thinker, seeking ways to comprehend biological puzzles in terms of pattern recognition. This attitude synthesized with Thomas Kuhn's vision of the successful scientist who is a passionate puzzle solver, who relishes the challenge to solve problems in which "the outcome remains very much in doubt."[24] Hard work and long hours of devotion were already the hallmark of Cerami's research and his psychological mainstay, and before the academic year began, he attended a summer course in biochemistry. It was here that he first met his future classmate, friend, and distinguished cell-biologist-to-be, Daniel Rifkin. Although Rifkin had already studied at Princeton, he recognized that the atmosphere at The Rockefeller University where students were treated like junior faculty was unique. As he recalled, "You were special, not students, more like junior colleagues. We had joined a guild. I liked Tony immediately, we were both from New Jersey, both interested in biochemistry and I could see that he was driven."[25]

On the day that the graduate program began, Cerami knew that a successful career in science would be contingent upon a great many variables. As he walked along 66th Street, he noticed a billboard advertising a new musical opening on Broadway: *Nowhere to Go but Up*. The show's title was to prove prophetic.

3 · THE SHAPING OF A SCIENTIFIC MIND

You're not really doing science unless you find yourself waking up in the middle of the night screaming.
— Gerald Edelman (in B. Ehrenreich, *Living with a Wild God: A Nonbeliever's Search for the Truth About Everything*)

The institute that Cerami entered in 1962 was a driving force of laboratory-centered investigation and one that made more major discoveries in biomedical science than any other research organization during the twentieth century.[1] Indeed, the history of the first biomedical institute in the United States is of global significance, for it was guided by a belief that health was fundamental to the improvement of the human condition. The Rockefeller Institute for Medical Research (RIMR) may have only occupied a small geographical space on the east side of the island of Manhattan, but it formed the centrifugal locus of an intricate network of investigators, institutions, investments, and influences that had a worldwide reach.

In order to fully understand the prodigious scientific achievements of the RIMR and how it molded Cerami's scientific attitude, we must first acknowledge the profound structural changes taking place in the United States at the end of the nineteenth century. A new plutocracy was emerging: the gilded titans of industrial capitalism, who had at their disposal such previously unimagined wealth that it enabled them to both conceive of, and seek to determine, the pace and direction of societal change. Of course, the United States had not been the first country to industrialize and to create a formerly unknown demographic category of industrial magnates. This had been achieved earlier in Britain, but many of the U.S. tycoons differed significantly from their British counterparts, who, in the main, had made philanthropic benefactions posthumously. For the new generation of industrial tycoons in the new world, human amelioration would be achieved through a program of vivid, proselytizing philanthropy. An outlier of this new sense of manifest duty was the steel magnate Andrew Carnegie, who in 1889 published an essay entitled *The Gospel of Wealth*. "The day is not far distant," Carnegie wrote, "when the man who dies leaving behind him millions of available wealth,

which was free for him to administer during life, will pass away unwept, unhon-
ored and unsung." This message of moral rectitude stuck a resonant chord with oil
millionaire and Baptist John D. Rockefeller Jr., who in the same year wrote a letter
to Carnegie announcing his conversion to the wisdom of actively initiating philanthropic programs to improve the human condition: "I would that more men of
wealth were doing as you are doing with your money but, be assured, your example will bear fruits and the time will come when men of wealth will more generally
be willing to use it for the good of others."[2]

In 1901, under the enlightened guidance of his adviser and fellow Baptist, Frederick Gates, John D. Rockefeller established the RIMR in adherence to his guiding economic philosophy, which he referred to as "the business of benevolence."[3]
Rockefeller, directed by passionate experts and advisers, helped to reconfigure the
role of U.S. philanthropy by establishing organizations that sought to address the
forces that had previously held back human well-being and development. Thus,
"the best philanthropy," according to Rockefeller, "involves a search for cause, an
attempt to cure evils at their source."[4] However, it is worth noting that the advent
of private foundations was not universally welcomed, and following the establishment of both the Carnegie Corporation and the Rockefeller Foundation, concerns
about how private resources were being spent in the name of the public good
prompted Congress' interrogation of foundations in 1915.[5] Without wishing to
overvalorize the relationship with Frederick Gates, John D. Rockefeller had one
of his most idealistic and effective adherents. Gates saw his role as that of a scientific statesman, and one of his early decisions was to appoint the physician-
scientist Simon Flexner as the first director of the RIMR. Flexner's remit was to
advance the new institute without restraint,[6] a role he performed assiduously until
1935. In terms of Flexner's influence on the direction of Rockefeller philanthropy
in general, it is worth remembering that he was a close personal friend of John D.
Rockefeller Jr. and was also the chairman of the Rockefeller Foundation. In fact,
all of the RIMR's directors after Flexner, through to Frederick Seitz (1968–1978),
simultaneously served as trustees of the Rockefeller Foundation. This close connectivity between the RIMR's researchers and the Rockefeller Foundation was to
prove of crucial importance in defining Cerami's later career and served to empha-
size how discoveries made in basic science at the RIMR could be rapidly translated into clinical use. In 1910, the Rockefeller Institute opened the first hospital in
the United States devoted entirely to patient-orientated research. Having a hospital on campus enabled the RIMR to maintain an unbroken spectrum of research,
from basic to clinical. From its earliest days, the hospital began to have an impact
on medical science and education; of the clinical scientists who were trained in the
hospital's first twenty-five years, more than one hundred went on to fill positions in
medical schools and hospitals in the United States and beyond. Throughout the
first half of the twentieth century, the RIMR pursued two central objectives: to
find innovative ways to understand human biology, both in health and disease,
while at the same time nurturing a new generation of young investigators. Both

ideals flourished under the presidency of Detlev Bronk, while his championing of the unity of science through international cooperation helped to link the remarkable contributions made to medicine within the fourteen acres on the island of Manhattan with the rest of the world.

The Rockefeller University was a truly inimitable institution, which for almost fifty years was able to operate entirely from the endowment provided by John D. Rockefeller Sr., and for Cerami, it seemed like the perfect place to pursue his life of scientific discovery. Located on the Upper East Side with a campus described rather lyrically by the *New York Times* as "a musical composition of light, shadow and shades of green," it provided housing for faculty and postdocs, an expansive medical library, and the intellectual freedom to pursue novel scientific ideas.[7] The academic course was what would be called today an open program, and while students were required to take one general class, there were no formal courses offered and no examinations. Bronk selected individuals on the criteria of self-motivation, and once chosen by The Rockefeller University, the idea of "being special" was imparted to such an extent that doctoral students began to think "Well . . . I had better be special."[8] As a graduate student, the mantra was "it doesn't matter whether you're first; you're going to have to be the best."[9] Such elevated expectations were not unrealistic: in the 1960s, The Rockefeller University was a remarkable place for Cerami's generation, who enjoyed advantages that no other student in the world could experience in terms of prestige, finance, and opportunity. Once accepted, it was incumbent upon each candidate to find a creative environment in which to follow their scientific interests. Cerami's research was carried out in the laboratory of Edward Tatum, a Nobel laureate in genetics,[10] under the direction of Edward Reich, a talented MD/PhD with a strong background in pharmacology. Over the next five years, Ed Reich offered the young researcher a self-styled "scientific buffet."[11] This variety encouraged Cerami to develop a proficiency in biochemistry, a readiness to discuss novel ideas, and a willingness to become a skilled experimenter in the laboratory. More than half a century later, when I visited Ed Reich at his home in Setauket, on the north shore of Long Island, he could still recall the task that he set Cerami in 1962: "the production of a synthetic DNA molecule which incorporated a changed structure designed to test the binding site of actinomycin to DNA." This was to be the subject of Cerami's PhD thesis and his first scientific paper.[12] The long hours of monotonous farm work undoubtedly helped to transform Cerami into a tenacious worker in the field of science as he set about exploring the task. As Reich noted, "Tony had an unbelievable capacity for work; there were not enough hours in the day for him."[13]

Cerami was Reich's first PhD student. His second, David Ward, arrived at The Rockefeller University via the University of Chicago and Harvard. All three men were gifted experimentalists, infused with a desire to make their mark in biomedical science, to create observations that other researchers could develop, and with energy to burn. Together, their exceptional and productive dynamic brought about what Ed Reich describes as "one of the most exciting moments that I've ever experienced in science."[14] Late one evening, the three experimenters gathered in the laboratory. Reich describes how they became captivated by the unfolding events:

> The moment of truth was to have arrived and that day Tony was supposed to prepare the polymer of the synthetic DNA which was to be tested. Once that was isolated we would be able to test it and establish whether we had succeeded or failed in a matter of minutes. To do this, Tony prepared the synthetic DNA and needed to dialyze it into a form which was compatible with the activity of the enzyme, but as it turned out, probably the dialysis bag had a perforation, and he lost the material that he was dialyzing and he had to go through the whole procedure again so that we could do the test. Because of this, the whole "day of truth" lasted well into the night. We eventually got to the point of doing the experiment at about 3 A.M. And the three of us were standing after the tests had been run, looking at the isotope counter to see what the result would be. Firstly, we ran several controls, and then came the key reaction to establish whether or not the actinomycin bound to the anticipated structure, and when that particular reaction product slipped into the isotope counter, we saw in an instant that the result had succeeded. The three of us embraced each other, and were dancing and kissing each other in the middle of the night. It was a moment that that could never be relived at any other time, and for Tony in particular, who had been working several years toward his thesis with no indication of whether he was making progress or not, because the whole idea rested on single reaction that was to be performed at the end of all his labor. Fortunately it worked out, so it was a wonderful moment. I've known several moments of that kind on other projects that I've worked on, but nothing quite like this, because the three of us were all involved physically. It was a time of great suspense, it was a memorable moment. I don't think any of us will ever forget it or probably anticipate such a moment again. It was like your first love.[15]

Cerami's middle of the night triumph was one small component of the broader evolution of the discipline of molecular biology that was occurring in the early 1960s. In the early decades of the twentieth century, advances in biochemistry and physiology gave rise to the idea that all living organisms are made up of lifeless molecules assembled to form cells and organs. Biochemistry described the complex pathways by which cells harness and utilize energy and how they are driven and controlled by numerous different chemical catalysts, or enzymes. Physiology, on the other hand, concerned itself with how the functions of groups of cells and organs are controlled and coordinated by hormones or reflex pathways in the nervous system, for example. It gradually became clear that all living processes can be studied, and to a large degree interpreted, by the methods and laws of chemistry and physics. That resulted in the emergence of a new science, molecular biology.[16] It was this new branch of biology, examining the structure and interactions of proteins and nucleic acids essential for life, that led Cerami, Ward, and Reich to collaborate on a project to isolate enzymes. With the discovery of enzymes at the end of the nineteenth century (derived from the Greek *en zume*, meaning "in yeast"), biochemistry arose as a new subfield of biology, concerned with the chemical nature of the various substances present in living cells and with the enzymes that make these substances and bring about these reactions.[17] Enzymes are highly specific, with each accomplishing one particular kind of chemical reaction. Along with their interest in enzymes, the researchers were similarly intrigued by another class of compounds also discovered at the end of the nineteenth century: the nucleic acids, given that their highest concentration is in the nucleus. These acids contain carbon, nitrogen, hydrogen, oxygen, and phosphorus. With enzymes and nucleic acids as their focus, the researchers found a successful personal alchemy based on mutual respect and a shared confidence in each other's skills at the bench, combined with a willingness to work to a punishing schedule. "It was an exciting time: we worked twelve to fourteen hours a day in the lab," remembered Dave Ward, "and at around 10 P.M. we would go up to First Avenue, a block away from the Rockefeller, and eat pizza, then back to the lab until midnight."[18] During the course of this intensive work, Cerami, Ward, and Reich developed a protocol for isolating a series of DNA and RNA polymerizing enzymes. The work constituted a significant experimental advance at the time.[19] Meanwhile, some of their other scientific activities were simply on too big a scale for the researchers to undertake at the Rockefeller laboratory. On one occasion, when they decided to prepare DNA polymerase from one ton (2,000 lbs) of *Escherichia coli*, they had to relocate to a facility in Boston, given that no enzymes were available from a commercial source. This laboratory had large vats that could accommodate 50 lbs of ammonium sulfate. Even so, the procedure compelled the three researchers to work in shifts to produce one large-scale preparation of DNA polymerase, which they would then crystallize, working with other scientific colleagues.[20]

Unlike many academic scientists who eschew forays into the uncertain world of business, even while still a PhD student, Cerami was the embodiment of the biomedical entrepreneur. Initially a role borne out of economic necessity, this work at the business–biology interface, while bringing considerable wealth, would also later give rise to destructive personal and commercial conflicts. Seeing that there was a commercial opportunity that could be exploited, Cerami, Reich, Ward, and a Rockefeller laboratory technician named Peter Leininger set up the company Biopolymers Inc. as a vehicle for their scientific dexterity. The need to augment their salaries was critical to the formation of the company, but no less acute was the desire to put a value on and to protect their scientific ingenuity. The need to protect one's intellectual property was uppermost in Cerami's mind from very early on in his career and was to form a cornerstone of his attitude relating to translational medicine (this attitude was contradicted by other scientists, who believed that it was their moral duty to challenge on both ethical and scientific grounds a model in which access to medical knowledge and treatments was controlled by commercial license agreements). Impoverishment, however, was not an aid to concentration, and Cerami was conscious of the dilemma that they faced:

"What we were doing was nucleic acid biochemistry, but in the '60s very few people had the enzymes and all the other things you needed to do this type of research. And people kept approaching us to give them reagents. It was the early days of molecular biology: DNA polymerase, RNA polymerase and all of the nucleotides—the molecular chunks that carry information in DNA and RNA. Initially we had felt obliged to give enzymes away for free, but we eventually decided that there might be a way to commercialize our work."[21] It was becoming rapidly apparent that they were part of the first wave of the molecular biology revolution, and just as they had wanted to know the mechanism by which actinomycin had killed bacteria, other researchers wanted to understand how their compounds worked at the molecular level. Crucially, this was at a time when individual scientists had to make their own reagents—the development of "off-the-shelf" preparations would be invaluable in terms of time savings.

The first step was to find premises for their embryonic biotech startup. It proved to be a far cry from the bespoke tabernacle of glass and chrome structures that now proliferate in science parks across many parts of the world. The laboratory of Biopolymers Inc. was housed in a former chicken coop on Cerami's parents' garden farm in New Jersey. Preparing the coop for the arrival of the state-of-the-art equipment demanded, according to Dave Ward, "the spirited shoveling of mounds of chicken manure."[22] Together, Cerami and Ward powered the company forward, working nonstop from Friday evening until Sunday evening on preparations of DNA polymerase, RNA polymerase, and various types of polymers that would then be put into the freezer. Cerami's father took the orders, packed them in dry ice, and shipped the preparations all over the world. Just how rarefied a service the company was providing was given troubling recognition when an FBI agent turned up at the farm to collect an order! Peter Leininger arranged to meet the FBI agent at the farm: when he handed over the refrigerated preparations, the government agent paid for the transaction with a cash-filled envelope. When Leininger asked what the FBI were going to do with the reagents, he was told that they were going to send the package to the Russians! In the aftermath of the 1962 Cuban Missile Crisis, the politics of the Cold War still dominated U.S.–Soviet relations, with the arch conservative Barry Goldwater, the five-time senator of Arizona, specializing in defense and foreign policy and Richard Milhous Nixon becoming the thirty-seventh president of the United States in 1969. There were two possible explanations as to why the American government was interested in the fledgling company. First, there was the possibility of reconfiguring the reagents for use in biological warfare. This was at a time when scientists were beginning to alter DNA by inserting plasmids—small circular molecules—and it was conceivable that the reagents would be necessary to change bacteria in order to put in a gene that would make some toxin. Second, an order may have been placed with Biopolymers Inc. that had originated in Russia, and the FBI thus felt compelled to investigate the company and examine their products. Once the FBI recognized that orders were going to both national and international destinations, and having seen the reassuring presence of Leininger and the converted chicken coop, their initial suspicions subsided. Nevertheless, it marked an extraordinary episode in the company's history.

While the existence of the business was in no way illegal or concealed, Cerami, wanting to give himself added kudos and an element of anonymity in the fledgling enterprise, assumed the pseudonym of Robert Kirk during the life of the enterprise: "I took on an alias because we talked to people who I didn't want to know I was a PhD student. So, I picked the name Kirk as it was my mother's maiden name." The company was a success, but eventually the grinding regime of working nonstop throughout the weekend became unsustainable, and the enterprise was sold to the Grand Island Biological Company (GIBCO) for what Dave Ward describes as "peanuts."[23] This is probably true, but all things are relative, and today Dave Ward, who is a member of the National Academy of Sciences, puts the realities of his first scientific enterprise into perspective: "We made about $10,000 apiece and my annual tuition stipend from The Rockefeller University in the 1960s was $2,200—so it turned out that it was very useful."[24] Beyond finances, Cerami and Ward formed a successful scientific partnership, both secure in their abilities and both demanding and driven. Tenacity was a shared personality trait, and it fashioned the basis of a strong friendship, which Cerami described in familial terms: "we were like two brothers, like two peas in a pod." The bold initiative would serve as a template for his future enterprises: as well as providing Cerami with much-needed cash at a time when his first child, Carla, was born, the experience of creating and running a biomedical startup company was at once educational and enticing, way beyond an economic expedient.

Back at The Rockefeller University, the institution's scientific structure epitomized what the parasitologist George Cross describes as "a German-type system composed of scientific fiefdoms,"[25] and this was certainly how it appeared to many of the graduate students in the 1960s. One of the new intakes joining Cerami was author and social commentator Barbara Ehrenreich (Barbara Alexander as she then was). In her beautifully crafted book *Living with a Wild God*, she recounts with consummate precision the scientific realities that existed in 1964: "The organization of lab work was, and still is, entirely feudal. A 'lab' was not only a place or a room or series of rooms, it was the fiefdom of a particular scientist. To 'go into' a lab as a grad student was to apprentice yourself to this scientist, with the idea that you would, after several years of patient toil, ascend to a similar rank yourself, at which point you would be able to offload the manual labor to people more junior than yourself."[26]

The Rockefeller University's central area of endeavor was biology, and soon after her arrival, Barbara Alexander joined the laboratory of the immunologist Gerald Edelman. Attracted by his "mad intensity," she recalls how "he told me and another potential student that you're really not doing science unless you find yourself 'waking up in the middle of the night screaming.'"[27] Alexander's entrance into Edelman's realm coincided with the summer of 1964 (Freedom Summer), and the changing social mores that were transforming society were not warmly embraced by Edelman. Far from it—in fact, on one occasion while dean of graduate studies, Edelman severely reprimanded the cell biologist Miki Rifkin when she was a student for having put up posters for a raunchy party, calling her to his office and informing her that "'that type of behavior was not going to be tolerated on campus.'"[28] The discrimination didn't end there; when Miki Rifkin was a graduate student, the underrepresentation of women was manifest; her class was made up of four women and twenty men, and there was not one single full professor at The Rockefeller University who was a woman.[29]

In 1962, the founding statement of the new left Students for a Democratic Society began: "We are people of this generation, bred in at least modest comfort, housed now in universities, looking uncomfortably to the world we inherit."[30] It was clear that by the 1960s, there was a growing and uncomfortable recognition that the postwar Truman–Eisenhower hegemony had run its course. For some, the Student Nonviolent Coordinating Committee's Freedom Summer Project inspired adherents in the early days of the new left, while young women involved in the civil rights movement began to openly question the dictates of patriarchy. As the counterculture was about to burst onto the wider social stage in a kaleidoscopic way, The Rockefeller University was not a hotbed of political unrest. Cerami and many of his friends remained immersed in discussing science in the Upper East Side of Manhattan rather than the politics of imperialism in Southeast Asia, something that would only change with the escalation of the war in Vietnam. Edelman remained allergic to the motives of the antiwar movement, and his suspicions led him to question the moral compass of even his Rockefeller colleagues. Edelman rejected the zeitgeist and warned Alexander that the politics of protest could lead to accusations of communism and that vigilance was needed at all times when associating with people from other labs because science was a competitive business, and the keeping of secrets was paramount.[31] Cerami was conscious of the siege mentality and wariness of kleptomania emanating from Gerald Edelman's lab: "Edelman's people weren't allowed to talk to others in case we would steal their ideas."[32] In fact, Edelman controlled his group so tightly that when he walked the corridors of the Institute, they were compelled to walk behind him rather like a prince with a trailing retinue.[33] There was, however, no doubting Gerald Edelman's scientific brilliance: his work uncovering the chemical structure of an antibody and how antibodies recognize the enormous number of toxins, bacteria, and other antigens encountered during a lifetime earned him the 1972 Nobel Prize in Physiology or Medicine, which he shared with the British biochemist Rodney Porter.

If the organization of science at The Rockefeller University was on a German model, then the social life of the university, especially the illustrious dining room, was quintessentially British in orientation. This owed much to the ideal of intellectual and social integration embodied by Oxford and Cambridge colleges, where eating at high table was seen as integral to the culture of learning. By engineering the mingling of individuals at lunch and dinner, the founders of The Rockefeller University believed that the frequent and intense interactions had the potential to change the way researchers viewed scientific problems and thereby minimize their tendency to make time-wasting mistakes. Certainly, while the gastronomy may have differed from Oxford and Cambridge, the eating of meals together while conversing about serious scientific matters was an important part of The Rockefeller University culture and an important means of integrating the scientific diversity and depth of the Institute.[34]

For Cerami, one of the most memorable aspects of life at The Rockefeller University was undoubtedly the lunch room, with its white linen tablecloths and dress code that necessitated the wearing of a jacket and tie for men or a dress for women. The food was deliberately prepared in a manner that was not so distractingly sumptuous that it detracted from the lively scientific discussions, which were the high point of the day. The atmosphere was one of ostentatious informality: everyone was expected to walk in and sit down next to senior and junior faculty members in whatever order they came into the room and then discuss science. This random seating configuration allowed Cerami to dine next to such scientific luminaries as Stanford Moore, Peyton Rous, Ed Tatum, Fritz Lipmann, Eugene Opie, and cell biologist George Palade. Palade, a Romanian American Nobel laureate, has been described as "the most influential cell biologist ever,"[35] and indeed, Cerami found Palade to be an inspiring teacher and an egalitarian and principled man openly interested in the ideas of others. The dining room was for Cerami an eminently conducive setting for provocative discussion, and critically, it was where he learned how to think scientifically: "I learned more in that dining room than in any didactic setting, just by watching how these people thought. A lot of them would ask what me what I was doing and this helped me explain my work by asking questions of myself. You learned on your feet—that was the important factor, and it was a scientifically inspiring setting."[36] Cerami was not alone in holding this belief. Nearly half a century earlier, his literary hero Paul de Kruif had also found the dining room one of the Institute's most stimulating characteristics: "At the lunch break there was balm for my discouragement. Here I could listen to the scintillating talk of my betters . . . I never tired of listening to the philosophy of Alexis Carrel, who had won the Nobel Prize in medicine . . . Carrel, who had been in America a long time, had carefully preserved his French accent, which made him sound to me even more learned than he was. . . . Then at the luncheon table there might be Dr Peyton Rous, refined, gentle, exquisitely cultured. . . . In this refectory there was an air of solemnity to be expected and appropriate to the unveiling of mysteries."[37]

For other researchers, perhaps those still grappling with the barely tractable complexities of human biology, it was with some trepidation that they entered the dining room. For them, rather than a place that sharpened their wits, it transmogrified into something of a medieval Star Chamber, where intellectual verdicts were handed down following the matter-of-fact query "and what is your molecule?"

British pathologist Siamon Gordon recalls one particularly intimidating encounter sitting on the bench seats and not knowing who was going to sit next to him: "One day Stanford Moore sat down beside me. Stanford was a lovely guy who later got the Nobel Prize with William Stein for discovering amino acid analysis. And he started the conversation by asking (and it was only lunchtime remember) 'what have you discovered today?'"[38] Nor were all the aristocrats of science entirely at ease while eating their lunch in such a hallowed setting. There were rumors that when mathematician, philosopher, and inventor of cybernetics Norbert Weiner occasionally entered the lunch room, people were so worried at the potential criticism of their work that there was a discernible movement out of the back door into the garden.[39] These golden days were not to last. The collegiate alchemy of the dining room was brought to an end during the era of financial retrenchment under the presidency of the physicist Fred Seitz, who succeeded Bronk in 1968. By the early 1970s, the changing economic environment brought about by industrial recession had begun to bite, providing the fiscal rationale for the dining room's closure. Over the preceding seventy years, it had been a nexus of integration and scientific communication. Although there were, to some, justifiable accusations of elitism, when it was replaced by a large impersonal cafeteria, the magical chemistry disappeared. For Cerami, The Rockefeller University "was never the same again."[40]

So complete was Cerami's devotion to science at The Rockefeller University that it precluded much of the external world from entering into his life in any meaningful way. The unspoken mantra of the laboratory was that you were serious and devoted to science, or you should not be there. This scientific exclusion zone came into sharp relief on Friday, November 22, 1963. Each Friday afternoon, a lecture took place in the domed Caspary Auditorium, the state-of-the-art building on The Rockefeller University campus that was an ideal forum for discussing the latest findings in cell biology and metabolic understanding. Traditionally, people met for tea before the lecture, but when Cerami tried to enter the main auditorium, he found a sign on the door that read "The President has been shot and the lecture has been cancelled." In subconscious disbelief, Cerami's first thought was, who would shoot Detlev Bronk? Then the full historical impact of the message became clear to the young researcher. With the assassination of John Fitzgerald Kennedy in Dallas, Texas, earlier that day, a new date, time, and place was anchored in Cerami's mind, tragically immortalized, never to be forgotten.

As the 1960s progressed, aspects of the decade's countercultural philosophies began to influence Ed Reich's lab. In 1964, another scientific idealist, Alan Kapuler, became Reich's third graduate student. Kapuler had been a brilliant undergraduate at Yale, where he graduated top of his class. Like many before him, he too had been inspired by Bronk to use his time at the Rockefeller to "learn as much as possible about science and to use that knowledge to serve humanity."[41] Eventually, Kapuler was to rebel against the conventional scientific career pathway and instead followed the wisdom of Bob Dylan and values of the counterculture enshrined in Timothy Leary's epochal phrase to "turn on, tune in, drop out." Today, Kapuler is a celebrated organic gardener and public domain plant breeder in Oregon, but in the 1960s, his meditations on scientific research contributed to the philosophical debates in the Reich laboratory about the role of science, its social utility, and how ideas pursued at the bench could be translated into treatments for patients. This was a technically fertile time for Cerami, who welcomed the permissive nature of the lab's scientific discourse. What was less welcome was the exponential growth in the number of graduates and postgraduate researchers with no corresponding expansion in working space. By the middle of the 1960s, as many as twelve to fourteen people were working in the 600-foot laboratory, making for an intense proximity that gave rise to discontent and occasionally some discord. The Rockefeller University's atmosphere of boiling ambition was played out in a confined, febrile atmosphere, where arguments about whether science was principally Baconian or, more unflatteringly, ignorance driven involved all of the researchers and no small amount of bravado. For David Ward, the conflicts that did occur were part of the natural order: "Ed was egotistical, so was Al, so was I and so was Tony. If you're a good scientist, you want to be acknowledged as being bright and smart, and that was the game of one-upmanship that we played."[42] During this period, Cerami was much more reserved than in later life, and when reflecting on the complexity of his character, he would candidly admit to being "not the easiest person to get along with," perhaps in part fueled by his early hunger for recognition.

A principal concept of the controlled scientific experiment is the removal of as many variables as possible, but such control is unimaginable when applied to the heterogeneous, free-floating intellects that inhabited Ed Reich's lab. Science is a collective endeavor after all, and there is a debate to be had as to whether the arc of its progress would move more quickly if its practitioners worked in concert or conflict. Vulgar vanities cannot always be camouflaged by an impenetrable layer of good manners and personal decorum, nor were Cerami's coworkers overburdened with a false sense of modesty: the laboratory was a Darwinian setting where real-life emotions were given full expression. In fact, the discussion as to whether The Rockefeller Institute for Medical Research should cultivate a consensus or conflict model went back to the scientific bloodlines of Paul de Kruif and his boss, Simon Flexner. In his memoir, de Kruif described his anger with Flexner over their different views of the Rockefeller staff and the goals of the Institute. De Kruif felt that having a central harmonious research family would be the death knell of any creative endeavor, suggesting that "all creating including science is a war against precedent. Science, to be vital, must grow out of competition between individual brains, foils one to the other, each man mad for his own idea."[43] Between Cerami and Dave Ward, there was plenty of interaction and much mutual respect, yet even so, the overpopulation of the lab led to a blurring of frontiers and the construction of demarcations between the two graduate students. "We had an eight-foot lab bench," Ward remembers, "and a line of adhesive tape dividing it. Mine was the right side and Tony's was the left side."[44] It was in those early years at The Rockefeller University that Cerami learnt that science is an all-consuming, self-directed profession.

In the summer of 1967, Cerami graduated with a PhD in biochemistry. He was twenty-six years old. The five years he had spent in New York had given him valuable insights into the natural world. He now understood that living things were mechanisms and wanted to use his knowledge of organic chemistry as a lens through which human biology could be understood. Seized with a sense of potential, Cerami looked around the world to see which institution would enable him to fulfill his ambition: to translate laboratory research into treatments for patients. He began his search at one of the world's oldest scientific institutions, the University of Oxford. Cerami's experience at the interview with Henry Harris for a postdoctoral position at the William Dunn School of Pathology did not match his expectations. Harris was a brilliant biologist, justly celebrated for his work on tumor suppressor genes, although arrogant and prone to demonstrations of his self-considered superior intelligence whenever possible. The William Dunn School's prowess in translational medicine was well known to Cerami, for it was there in 1941 that the therapeutic discovery of penicillin had been made by Howard Florey and his team. However, on being shown around the august institution, Cerami realized that if he took the job, he would be worked relentlessly with little hope of advancing his knowledge of the subjects that fascinated him the most: medicine and the pathogenic mechanisms of disease. Cerami's teenage conviction that the diseases he witnessed on the family farm could shed light on the causes of human disease set him on a path that was to be his life's work. Not that he wanted to be a clinician dealing directly with patients: it was the pathology and pathogenesis of disease that captivated him. Inherently, Cerami felt that his science should have a practical utility, and equally he recognized that he lacked a modern understanding of disease processes that would be necessary to develop new therapies. Seemingly, there was no alternative: if he was going to develop a biomedical ideation, he needed to enroll in some courses at a medical school.

During his graduate training, Cerami had spent one year working on a collaborative project in the laboratory of the pharmacologist Irving Goldberg at Harvard.[45] Goldberg and Ed Reich had been on the House Staff at Columbia University Medical Center together in the 1950s, and both were determined to do all that they could to find Cerami a place at Harvard Medical School. In the summer of 1967, however, the biggest impediment to joining Harvard's histology and pathophysiology classes was the limited number of complete sets of slides for the course, which was capped at 100. At the time, Goldberg was an associate professor and did not think he possessed the necessary influence with the administration's hierarchy, so he approached his boss, Howard Hiatt, Blumgart Professor of Medicine at Harvard Medical School. Possibly there may have been an extra set of slides kept under lock and key, or conceivably someone dropped out of the course, or more likely Hiatt's powers of persuasion triumphed: Cerami was allowed to attend the Harvard Medical School as a special student for one year.[46]

Cerami came from a lab where good ideas counted and were taken seriously, but ideas are cheap unless they are capitalized upon. Conviction in itself will not make a scientist, but you would be hard-pressed to become one without it. Very early on, Cerami came to the realization that if he was going to add to the knowledge of disease treatment, then he would first have to fathom some of the mysteries of human biology, and so at Harvard, he sought out medical exposure as a means to advance his understanding of the prevention and treatment of disease. As he later wrote,

> This was an incredible experience. Not only did I learn about medicine, but I also spent my spare time in the library reviewing the literature concerning the pathophysiology of cachexia, as well as the current understanding of the cause of diabetic complications. I formulated an outline of how to approach each of these entities using the available knowledge. There were of course, various theories put forward to explain these phenomena, but each lacked experimental proof. Various mediators were suggested to be responsible for cachexia, and diabetic complications were thought to be due to elevated glucose levels that stimulated the biosynthesis of glycoproteins in susceptible tissues.[47]

Cerami's experiences at Harvard put him at the vanguard of translational medicine, a field rapidly evolving thanks to a combination of experimental procedures, new instruments, and the efforts of pioneering scientists working in the United States and beyond. Another Rockefeller graduate interested in the pathology and pathogenesis of disease was the immunologist Barry Bloom, and while neither researcher was a qualified physician, they were probably more focused on specific diseases than many clinicians.[48] Both were concerned with the medical application of their research and committed to bringing the knowledge and methods of innovative basic science to alleviate the burden of human diseases. A research methodology had been evolved by Cerami: to understand the mechanism of disease as a pathway to discovering efficacious treatment. Paradoxically, being a chemist rather than a physician turned out to be an advantage. Working outside his own discipline, Cerami was unencumbered by the conventions that inevitably build up over time within any field. He thus remained free to use his imagination to solve nature's puzzles: indeed, as Charles Darwin had related a century before, "no one could be a good observer without being an active theorizer."[49] It was at Harvard that Cerami's distinctive approach began to crystallize in his own mind, with the realization that he could apply his chemical knowledge to biology. This laid the foundation for Cerami's approach to seeking treatments for disease, as one of his intuitive abilities was postulating theories, what he termed "pattern recognition" in biological systems, which steered him toward seeing immunology as chemical reactions between molecules.

Life in Boston was sublime: the science was liberating and the Cerami family lived in a comfortable apartment in Roslindale, with evenings and weekends spent walking in the bucolic setting of the Arnold Arboretum. The year passed quickly, and now with the fruits of his medical training shaping his research methodology, Cerami continued his biomedical education with a postdoctoral fellowship at the Jackson Laboratory in Bar Harbor, Maine. Under the influence of the immunologist George Snell, who won the Nobel Prize in 1980,[50] the Jackson Laboratory in the 1960s was the world's leading institution for mouse genetics. Cerami was immediately attracted to the work of two of the laboratory's biochemists: Andrew Kandutsch, who studied histocompatibility antigens, and Douglas Coleman for his insights into the role of genetics in the severity of diabetes in mice.[51] Coleman was a warmhearted and kind friend and a visionary biochemist, establishing the then heretical finding that genetics could control obesity.[52] Witnessing Doug Coleman's courageous stance against accepted thinking proved a valuable lesson for Cerami later in his career, giving him the fortitude to stay true to his own scientific beliefs and march against the consensus. At weekends, Coleman would arrange visits to nature reserves on the coast of Maine for Cerami and his family, which gave his toddler son Tom the opportunity to play with Tony's daughter Carla. Levitations like this aside, it is hard to imagine a further cry from Cerami's vision of "the good life" than his year spent at the Jackson Laboratory. No amount of cognitive dissonance could camouflage the sense that he felt geographically isolated and desperately missed metropolitan cultural life and its heady mix of amplified ambition and limitless potential. A sense of spiritual torpor swirled around him during the dark winter months of 1969. Relief from his social and cultural dislocation came in a familiar form. Throughout his life, Cerami felt a need to be in control, to navigate his own life journey, and in 1969, temporarily at least, salvation was secured when he returned to The Rockefeller University, the citadel of basic research, as an assistant professor in his own laboratory of experimental hematology. The scientific connective tissue had been regenerated, and from that moment, Cerami realized that the laboratory was his natural habitat. Like many of his scientific idols had done before him, he would surely stay at The Rockefeller University forever. Surely. . . .

4 · THE ROCKEFELLER UNIVERSITY AND THE BROAD HORIZON

Tony Cerami always had an eye on disease treatment.

—Sir John Bell (interview, April 2016)

In terms of the social context in which translational science takes place, an important literary allegory for Cerami's early career can be found in Sinclair Lewis's book *Arrowsmith*, published in 1925 and which was probably the first significant American novel to concern itself with the culture of science.[1] In the book, the eponymous Martin Arrowsmith is an idealist: his goal is to be a research scientist who discovers the mysteries of biology and the causes of human diseases. The pinnacle of his life, where Arrowsmith feels that he is making the greatest contribution to medicine, occurs when he becomes a medical researcher at the McGurk Institute, which is modeled on the Rockefeller Institute. His mentor Max Gottlieb shares with him what it is to be a scientist: "The scientist . . . will not accept quarter-truths, because they are an insult to his faith."[2] Where science was treated as religion, absolute proof, intellectual discipline, and rigorous experimentation were the researcher's sole catechism and the foundations of Cerami's work ethic that had been established under the tutelage of Tatum and Reich.[3] Untested dogma was anathema, and The Rockefeller University provided the perfect environment for the early career Cerami to explore the boundaries of translational medicine with freedom and vigor. If, as Cerami believes, it was his teacher Mr. White who had given him his scientific life and had done so without ostentation and free of any thought other than a devotion to his profession, it was The Rockefeller University that gave him the resolve to believe in his own ideas. The Rockefeller University's ideal of a laboratory-without-walls encouraged him to develop a boundary-hopping, cross-disciplinary approach, a kind of modern-day elastic thinking that enabled him to extemporize a way forward and explore the living world. Cerami had eclectic interests, and pulling together information from different fields was to become his distinctive strategy.[4]

His science was guided by a sense of idealism: the belief that science should have a social utility and an overwhelming personal drive to alleviate the human suffering caused by disease. But where to start—what would provide the scientific roadmap for his journey in translational medicine? He decided that the most fruitful way forward was to understand the basic mechanisms of what was going on in the human body and then to discover ways to better diagnose and treat diseases. It was this interface between diagnosis and treatment that was the ground he was determined to occupy. This curiosity-driven discovery research led Cerami to anemia—a deficiency of hemoglobin in the blood—that was an underlying cardinal symptom of some of the diseases that he hoped to investigate. This, in turn, directed him to erythropoietin (EPO), a peptide hormone produced in the kidney that acts on the bone marrow to stimulate blood cell production. Cerami was highly proficient at protein isolation, and it was with monomaniacal concentration that he set about isolating EPO from the urine of anemic patients. Working with a female patient with aplastic anemia at the Rockefeller hospital, Cerami collected her urine for over a year and concentrated it in his laboratory. Frustratingly, the urine still contained other proteins, particularly albumin—a major protein of blood—which, being a glycoprotein, had many kinds of sugar groups attached. Recognizing that the existing technology was deficient, after two long years of unsatisfying experiments in the lab, Cerami admitted defeat and gave up the project to isolate EPO.[5] This initial foray into translational research left him feeling depressed and discouraged;[6] temperamentally, he was ill-suited to failure, a characteristic that proved both his strength as well as his weakness.[7] Nevertheless, although it was not readily apparent at the time given the seeming disappointments of the project, investigating the role of EPO in human physiology marked one of the truly decisive moments in Cerami's career in translational medicine: the steps taken here at The Rockefeller University early in Cerami's working life would become the foundations of a return to the EPO molecule forty years later.

While working on EPO, Cerami also began to investigate ways to treat an array of rare diseases, including cystic fibrosis, sickle cell disease, thalassemia, and hemophilia—what Cerami, with his gift for taxonomy, came to describe as "orphan diseases."[8] A central feature uniting of all these diseases was their unmet clinical need: pharmaceutical companies, whose raison d'être was making a profit rather than curing disease, were economically disinterested in finding cures for rare diseases. Conversely, this neglected status was exactly what attracted Cerami to their amelioration: "There was nothing being done for people with orphan diseases. Pharmaceutical companies didn't want to know, so that was why I decided to be there in that space. I thought we might get lucky and come up with something useful."[9] An early candidate for investigation was thalassemia, a genetic disorder of hemoglobin synthesis.[10] A major feature of the disease is severe anemia, and a principal physiological problem associated with anemia is that its treatment requires repeated blood transfusions, which in turn create a further complication—the accumulation of iron in the patient. Iron is necessary for oxidative metabolism, but iron overload is life threatening, with the substance often aggregating in the heart, leading to cardiac disease and early death. Meanwhile, the toxic effects of the condition can also afflict the pancreas.[11] By the beginning of the 1970s, Cerami had designed a research project with the aim of finding an iron-chelating agent that, when taken orally, would travel through the body capturing the excess iron before safely being expelled in the patient's urine. The next step was to find a postgraduate assistant skilled in chemistry who shared Cerami's imaginative appetite for science and what American theoretical physicist Richard Feynman described as "the kick in discovery."

Salvation came in the form of a phone call from Hans Fisher, professor of nutritional biochemistry at Rutgers University. Fisher alerted Cerami to the skills of a talented PhD student, Joseph Graziano, who had just graduated and was in need of an academic job. A week later, on Friday, November 26, 1971, the day after Thanksgiving, Graziano attended an interview and subsequently became Cerami's first postdoctoral student on a salary of $8,000. For Joe Graziano, the early years spent in Cerami's lab defined the arc of his scientific career and provided him with space to learn to think creatively and to overcome the imposter syndrome that many research workers had experienced upon entering the hallowed corridors of The Rockefeller University. It was of course a formidable environment that demanded intellectual persistence, self-belief, and no small amount of sacrifice. Graziano vividly remembers that "Tony was relentless in his creativity, he would come up with a dozen ideas every day. We would work until 10 P.M.—I had two children—and when I eventually got home the phone would ring around 11.15 P.M. It would be Tony wanting to talk about the latest experiment."[12]

Throughout the 1970s, Cerami, often with Joe Graziano,[13] contributed to the understanding of iron metabolism and hematopoiesis in thalassemia and directed a more focused approach to iron chelation therapy.[14] But to take a drug from the laboratory to application in patients is a scientifically complex and emotionally demanding undertaking. Cerami's disease-focused research did not always have an immediate chemotherapeutic impact, something that, on occasion, led to his emotional desolation. During this period, there were only three people working in the lab: Tony, the laboratory technician James Leong, and Joe Graziano. Such close proximity removed any prospect of camouflaging inner emotions, and Graziano witnessed the effect that experimental setbacks had on his mentor: "Tony was the smartest person I've ever met, hands down. Full of enthusiasm, but he can be manic and depressive, and [on occasion] could get very melancholic."[15] The disheartening feelings associated with multiple unsuccessful outcomes can be overwhelming, especially after the investment of considerable time and effort. Paradoxically, while there was no escaping Cerami's inability to successfully isolate EPO or to discover a truly effective iron-chelating drug, in retrospect, these failures revealed an important truth. Some of the defining discoveries of Cerami's career came as a result of failures in other research projects, perhaps most notably the discovery of TNF while seeking a treatment for African sleeping sickness, or the breakthrough with HbA1c while unsuccessfully searching for a treatment for sickle cell disease. Failures, irrespective of their short-term negative tone, were often essential experiences on the path to important discoveries.[16] Very soon Cerami's Laboratory of Experimental Hematology had built a reputation for drug development, propelled by a belief in persistence and that possessing an "off-center way of thinking," unconfined by the accepted orthodoxy, could be a valuable pathway to finding new insights into the cause and treatment of disease.[17]

Just how scientifically open-minded and unconventional Cerami was during this period became apparent when he welcomed (at least initially) into his lab the Swiss physician-scientist Ernst Friedheim as a guest professor and investigator. The Swiss, a pioneer in the field of chemotherapy, had studied physical chemistry and cell biology at The Rockefeller Institute for Medical Research in 1930. Friedheim may have been in his eightieth year, but Cerami rejected ageist stereotyping and hoped that by some process of scientific osmosis, the qualities that had led Friedheim to develop Mel B (melarsprol) for the treatment of African sleeping sickness and other drugs for chelation therapy of mercury and lead poisoning would infuse imaginative chemotherapeutic thinking in his lab. He was not disappointed. Friedheim was eccentric, brilliant, and inspiring, and being independently wealthy was not a financial burden on the laboratory's scarce resources. Joe Graziano had developed a passion for drug development from Cerami, and while working with Friedheim on the development of chelating compounds, he recognized a symmetry between the two researchers' scientific attitudes: "Ernst was like another version of Tony, he was constantly asking people, 'so, what's your molecule?' We immediately started to work developing one of Ernst's diethyl compounds as a chelating agent for lead. It proved to be a life-altering collaboration."[18] In the laboratory, the compound was shown to successfully chelate lead in animals and caused elimination in the body via urine.[19] Despite Friedheim's death from kidney cancer in New York in 1989 at the age of eighty-nine,[20] Graziano continued the research work, and in 1991, their orphan drug was approved for use in patients. The treatment has proved so effective against lead poisoning—lead affects haem synthesis—that in 2014, the Friedheim–Graziano drug (2,3-dimercaptosuccinic acid) was listed as number 66 on the World Health Organization's list of essential medicines. It had been almost four decades since the publication of the first scientific paper on the efficacy of the compound: time-consuming years of seeming obscurity before the work was accorded proper recognition, years when it would have been all too easy to have given up along the way. More than anything, the episode is a valuable illustration of the value of persistence, something that Graziano attributes to the tremendous early career influence of Cerami, who taught him "not to give up on your molecule until it flames out."[21]

It is worth remembering that in the early years of Cerami's life as an independent researcher, most investigators at The Rockefeller University were primarily interested in very basic research rather than clinical research. One of his colleagues at the time was Rene Dubos, the French biologist and ecologist. Dubos was known for claiming that the most important advances come from individuals who stray from obvious paths and venture into unexplored areas. "It is not easy," he said, "to integrate these temperamental trailblazers into the rigid and cumbersome structure of large educational and research institutions."[22] This capacity and freedom to blaze a new path was given added impetus when Cerami was granted his own laboratory in a subterranean space in the Smith building, named in honor of the microbiologist Theobald Smith. Smith, described by Paul de Kruif as "the captain of American microbe hunters,"[23] was one of the pioneers whose investigations had inspired the teenage Cerami. In 1884, Smith and his veterinarian colleague F. L. Kilbourne were tasked by the U.S. Congress and the Bureau of Animal Industry to seek a remedy for Texas fever, a debilitating cattle disease that threatened the emergent beef industry and was costing the economy $60 million a year, or about $1.2 billion in today's value.[24] In their formal report published in January 1893, considered a masterful example of scientific method and clarity of logic, they revealed that the cause of Texas fever in cattle was the tick-borne protozoan parasite *Babesia bigemina*. The study was a marvelous piece of medical detective work, but its importance went far beyond solving the mystery of Texas fever. Smith and Kilbourne had described an entirely new means for a disease to pass between one host and another. It moved via a type of delivery service, through a vector—a tick—and the migration was complicated, involving the interlocking of three life cycles: that of the pathogen, the vector, and the host. This work primed the field for other vector-borne discoveries: malaria and mosquitoes, African sleeping sickness and the tsetse fly, and bubonic plague via rats and fleas.[25] The often acerbic de Kruif showed unqualified admiration for Smith's microbe-hunting proficiency: "He loved Beethoven, did young Smith, and for me this 'Investigation into the Nature, Causation, and Prevention of Texas or Southern Cattle Fever' has all the quality of that Eighth Symphony of Beethoven's sour later years. Absurdly simple in the working out of these themes—just as nature is at once simple and finitely complex. . . . And so, with this report, Theobald Smith made mankind turn a corner, showed men an entirely new and fantastic way a disease may be carried—by an insect."[26]

Following in Smith's footsteps, and with Smith's name emblazoned on his new laboratory, Cerami too was turning a corner. He had succeeded in navigating the difficult early years of his professional career and was beginning to attract research grants from outside sources together with graduate students of exceptional aptitude. Underpinning this burgeoning reputation was a distinctive attitude: Cerami's strength as a translational scientist was that he was not a specialist. Rather, he deliberately sought a wide-ranging perspective in order to gain a better understanding of human biology in both disease and health. The "broad horizon" was his vantage point, as the broader the thought process, the better, given that one never knew "where the insights [were] going to come from."[27] The broad-horizon, cross-discipline approach to biomedical investigation gradually brought recognition within the scientific community and led Cerami to develop a wide spectrum of scientific interests, including diabetes, orphan diseases, nutrition, and the science of food, or what is termed today "gastrophysics."[28]

Much of this scientific amplitude was informed by the familial and agricultural world that Cerami came from, a milieu that led him to develop wide-ranging interests that would be sustained throughout the length of his career. Both within and away from the lab at The Rockefeller University, his diverse expertise was often foregrounded by intriguing social contexts. On a macro level, the Rockefeller Foundation had long-standing interests in agriculture, agronomy, crop improvement, and nutrition since the 1930s, culminating in 1970 with the Nobel Peace Prize awarded to the foundation's Norman Borlaugh in recognition of his work modernizing agriculture in low-income countries: an effort popularly known as the Green Revolution. However, on a more immediate level, for Cerami and some of his colleagues, New York City was far removed from the green-hued farmers markets that flourish in parts of the city today. In 1974, the streets around The Rockefeller University were a desert for fresh fruit and vegetables, and it was only in the thinly spread satellite of local shops that vegetables of any sort could be sourced. The Ceramis together with David and Barbara Luskutoff and ten other families on The Rockefeller University campus faced a real dilemma—how to provide a balanced nutritional diet for their children? This deleterious situation had echoes of the ecological concerns of the author Jane Jacobs, who in 1961 published her influential work *The Death of the Great American Cities*. Jacobs—in a similar vein to Rachel Carson's highly influential book *Silent Spring*, published a year later—brought environmental concerns to the American public in a very direct way. A proselytizer and tireless campaigner, Jacobs was a vociferous opponent of Robert Moses, the all-powerful planner who transformed New York in the decade after World War II with the most intensive public construction program in the city's history. Jacobs was a native New Yorker and saw modernization as fundamentally misanthropic, suggesting instead that cites should be characterized by different shops and activities that would make life more livable, modeled on a human scale. Her concern had a resonance and foreshadowed present-day criticism of planners' willing sacrifice of cities to the car in the mid-twentieth century. Ironically, it was the motorcar that was the salvation to the paucity of fresh fruit and green vegetables in the immediate environs of The Rockefeller University.

The twelve health-conscious, liberal-minded families decided to form a co-op to make weekly excursions to the vast Hunts Point Wholesale Food Market in the Bronx. The only limiting factor was that so few of the co-op members owned an automobile, but with some effort and pooled resources, three vehicles were made available for the early morning trips north to the largest food distribution center in the world. Unsurprisingly, with the vegetable co-op containing so many experimental scientists, a great deal of planning went into its form and function. All twelve families paid a weekly subscription of $10, and every week, two people, a driver and gatherer from different families, made the 5:30 A.M. journey from York Avenue through some of the city's northern rundown, red-light, neighborhoods to

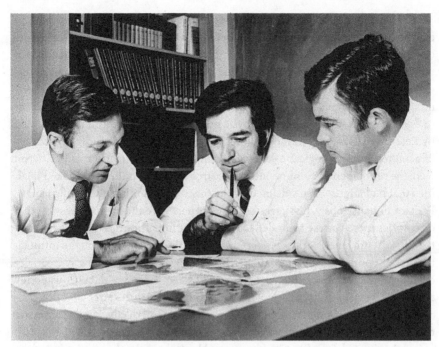

From left to right: Peter N. Gillette, Anthony Cerami, and James M. Manning. The team worked on sickle cell anemia at The Rockefeller University. Circa 1970.

Hunts Point. Twice a month, Tony would walk three blocks across The Rockefeller University campus to meet Barbara Luskutoff, who would then drive her station wagon off into the early rumble of the morning traffic. All twelve of the families in the co-op agreed upon one thing: Tony Cerami knew his onions! "My agricultural background," recalls Cerami, "allowed me to be able to select the best seasonal produce available and we would then fill the station wagon to overflowing!"[29] This matter-of-fact recollection belies the often intimidating, febrile atmosphere of the market, populated as it was by sleep-deprived truck drivers, warehouse men, and time-pressed retail merchants jostling shoulder to shoulder to secure the most competitive prices. This tumultuous setting was far removed from the polite collegiate haven of The Rockefeller University, but for Barbara Luskutoff, the bimonthly shopping expeditions with Cerami were captivating. "We had fun, and because the market was very macho and verbal, Tony was always there as my protector. You needed a strong person to get the best prices, luckily Tony knew the scene and how to handle things, that is why it worked so well."[30] Inevitably, on occasion, Cerami would buy great bushels of produce that were so mysterious and rare that his fellow co-operators were confused as to what they were or indeed how to cook them! However, the Rockefeller vegetable co-op was a beautifully conceived system that worked well and helped to bind the separate families together in the holistic fashion envisaged by Jane Jacobs.

Back in the laboratory, Cerami's work at the "broad horizon" continued to expand his understanding of the pathogenesis of disease and of ways to translate discovery into drugs and diagnostic tests. Indistinguishable from the substance of this research was the *method* of acquiring the necessary knowledge to make discovery possible. It was the fine-tuning of this scientific method that made Cerami's early professional years at The Rockefeller University so pivotal to his later career and that resonated deeply with the philosophy of scientific inquiry outlined by Peter Medawar, who in 1960 had received the Nobel Prize for the discovery of acquired immunological tolerance. For Medawar, imagination and criticism were the fundamental components of research and were much overlooked qualities that had largely been sidelined by the format of traditional scientific papers. Perhaps unconsciously, he suggested, most papers gave the false impression that discoveries merely arose from deductive observation. They did not make it clear that the essential mental process in research was the imaginative act, the formulation of a hypothesis to be tested later by experiments. For Medawar, creativity occupied the central position in the nature of scientific thought. What was truly telling was an inspiration, a flash of insight.[31] Cerami's early research on EPO, thalassemia, and orphan diseases met Medawar's criteria perfectly. While successful outcomes may not have been as immediate or as dazzling as he had hoped, the blaze of imagination to bring about "the conceptual breakthrough," the creative use of the broad horizon, and the persistence required to see the work through were all to become the defining characteristics of his life scientific.[32] Perhaps most significantly, Cerami realized early on that most scientific breakthroughs arrived in unexpected ways. It was his ability to see biological connections that others could not that formed the hinge upon which his career turned. As the geneticist Sir John Bell has observed, "The fun is seeing something for the first time, something that no one else has spotted and pursuing it."[33]

5 · DIABETES
The Creation of the Hemoglobin A1c Test

You can see a lot just by looking.
—Yogi Berra, American professional baseball catcher

On occasion, failure can be the harbinger of innovation, and for those who learn from their disappointments and persevere with the life scientific, new insights arising from experiments can lead to unexplored, unexpected, and exciting new understanding of disease processes and treatments.[1] For Cerami, just such a moment resulted from his failure to find a new treatment for patients with sickle cell disease: he survived the feelings of intense disappointment by holding tightly to his vision that science should be used to make the world a better place. Propelled forward by two imperatives, the belief that he could help people and the excitement of discovery, Cerami utilized the ideas, observations, and discoveries made during his investigations of sickle cell disease to discover a new diagnostic test, hemoglobin A1c (HbA1c), that has become a foundation for the treatment and diagnosis of diabetes across the world.

The HbA1c story begins at a cocktail party for a group of hematologists in New York City in 1971.[2] Cerami attended this meeting, and over daiquiris and martinis, he was told by one of the participants that there had been a recent report of the successful treatment for sickle cell anemia in patients by the administration of large amounts of urea (also known as carbamide).[3] The rationale given by the researchers was that the urea would disrupt hydrophobic bonds between the hemoglobin S molecules and allow the trapped sickled cells to progress through the capillaries.[4] To Cerami, a scientific investigator who looked at biology from a chemist's perspective,[5] this explanation seemed implausible as such a transition would require physiologically unfeasible high concentrations of urea.[6] In fact, to administer a disrupter of hydrophobic bonds in such concentrations would crystallize the patient!

However, more biologically persuasive to Cerami was the possibility that the clinical effects could be the result of the carbamylation of hemoglobin S with cyanate because urea in solution is in equilibrium with ammonium and cyanate ions. The finding that urea solutions were in equilibrium with cyanate that could react with proteins had been first observed with the enzyme ribonuclease.[7] Working with James Manning and Martha Fedorko, Cerami was able to demonstrate that cyanate could react with the amino terminal valines of hemoglobin S and prevent the sickling of cells following deoxygenation in vitro[8] and in vivo.[9] The question now was whether this observation could be translated from the laboratory bench into a therapeutic use with sickle cell patients. Cerami was beginning to make a name for himself as an applied scientist who took basic science discoveries and immediately translated them into clinical use.[10]

Hemoglobin is the protein inside red blood cells responsible for transporting oxygen from the lungs around the body to tissues and organs. All of the hemoglobin disorders are Mendelian recessive, meaning that for someone to present with the disease, they must inherit the gene from both parents. The atypical hemoglobin S distorts the red blood cells into the eponymous "sickle" or crescent shape that induces them to aggregate together, producing great pain, and their premature destruction can lead to chronic anemia and strokes.[11] With such a dystopian prognosis, it was no wonder that Cerami was entirely dedicated to finding a treatment to ameliorate the biological fate of sickle cell patients. The progression of his thinking and the biochemical reasoning informing his actions are penetrating: "I changed some sickle cells from a patient and put them under deoxygenating conditions and they would sickle but if you reacted them first with small amounts of cyanate, then they didn't. So the carbamylation of the amino terminal of ayalene was enough to prevent polymerization from occurring. So, I thought, well, we know urea is a natural product, it is found in all of us, we are all carbamylated to some degree, what we are doing is giving a little bit more so why don't we give it to sickle cell patients? And so we started to give cyanate to sickle cell patients. We gave cyanate to animals and showed that with amounts that were reasonable it wasn't really that toxic. So we started to do clinical studies, in those days the FDA was quite lenient compared to today and we had permission, and we gave the treatment, and we could show that there was less sickling of the blood and the hemoglobins went up and they had less crisis. Very quickly I became known for this work on hemoglobin S."[12]

There is no escape from the axiom that every new treatment of a disease must be assessed on patients suffering from that disease, and the early indications gave rise to optimism. The reaction of sodium cyanate with hemoglobin S prevented cells from sickling, reduced the anemia, and prevented crises in patients.[13] But, within two years, confidence in the treatment rapidly evaporated, as exposure to cyanate began to show debilitating side effects. Several patients unfortunately developed subcapsular cataracts and peripheral neuropathy similar to that seen in diabetics. Fortunately, these changes among the patients disappeared within a few months of cessation of the drug. That the long-term use of cyanate was obviously not a viable option for the treatment of sickle cell disease had a demoralizing impact on Cerami. He was thirty-one years old, and his first attempt to translate a treatment from the controlled laboratory setting to patients who suffered from the disease had ended in failure.

To some extent, his disappointment was tempered by the knowledge that the treatment had relieved the patients from many of the effects of the disease. Unquestionably, one of Cerami's defining scientific strengths is his ability to think creatively, outside the consensus—but the use of cyanate to treat patients was viewed skeptically by some physician-scientists working in the field of inherited blood disorders. One of the world's leading hematologists and Cerami's good friend, Sir David Weatherall, is a dissenting voice: "I think that it was looked upon as a bit of a joke in our field. The last thing you want to do is start treating your patients with poison. And my colleague and former boss at Johns Hopkins, Victor McKusick, had severe doubts; he thought that pouring cyanate into humans was a bit risky."[14]

Sitting on a battered sofa in the confines of his lab in the Theobald Smith Building, three floors below street level, Cerami felt an intense sense of discouragement about the direction of his research.[15] A generation earlier, the celebrated American educationalist, Abraham Flexner, recognized that the path of research is often unpredictable, that the pursuit of knowledge for its own sake is laudable, and that time spent on an investigation that does not bring immediate impact is not wasted. Flexner was the author of the Flexner Report in 1910, which led to the reform of medical education in the United States. He was also the brother of Simon Flexner, who was one of the founders of The Rockefeller University (formally The Rockefeller Institute). Abraham Flexner was adamant in his belief that the cultivation of curiosity at institutions of learning was the most likely way of contributing to human welfare. In his famous 1939 essay *The Usefulness of Useless Knowledge*, he argued that the most powerful technological, medical, and intellectual advances usually emerged from research that initially appeared useless without much relevance to real life. "Curiosity, which may or may not eventuate in something useful, is probably the outstanding characteristic of modern thinking. It is not new. It goes back to Galileo, Bacon and Sir Isaac Newton, and it must be absolutely unhampered."[16] Most scientific breakthroughs arrive in unexpected ways, and it was Cerami's ability to stretch his own brain and to see connections that others could not that was an exemplar of his resilience.

In the early 1970s, most biochemists were trained in terms of enzymologically catalyzed reactions; what was unusual about Cerami was that he was fascinated by reactions that can happen between small molecules and biological systems that were not enzymatically catalyzed. Indeed, once the dejection from the cyanate experiment had eased, Cerami was able to think more clearly and recognized that far from leading him up a blind alley, the investigation had uncovered a significant scientific discovery. In conversations with ophthalmologists and neurologists, both noted that the cyanate-induced harm was similar to that seen in diabetes. This had a catalyzing effect and reminded Cerami of two reports,[17] of patients with diabetes having an increased amount of the minor hemoglobin A1c.[18] The structure was unknown but appeared to be attached to the amino terminus of the beta chain of hemoglobin—exactly the same place where cyanate reacts. This was a eureka moment for Cerami, which led him to hypothesize, "Jesus, HbA1c was some sugar-like thing that was a chemically reactive compound in the blood of diabetics that could react with hemoglobin to form hemoglobin A1c and with other body proteins to explain the pathogenesis of diabetic complications."[19] As previously noted, Cerami was alerted to HbA1c by a paper written by Samuel Rahbar, a clinician working with his friend, the renowned hematologist Helen Ranney at the Albert Einstein College of Medicine. However, Rahbar only wrote two research papers on HbA1c, the first in 1968 while he was at the University of Tehran. The main focus of Rahbar's work was the identification of mutant hemoglobins, not A1c. Therefore, while Cerami was not the first researcher to discover HbA1c, he was certainly the first to understand its significance and that it held out the possibility of being used to give an integrated blood-glucose concentration for a previous period of time.

Cerami had been curious about diabetes since childhood when he saw many members of his mother's family suffer and die from the disease. In fact, his mother, Hazel, developed type 2 diabetes, and this motivated him to gain an understanding of the mechanism of the disease and, if possible, develop a therapy that might be helpful to patients.[20] For Cerami, the important factor was the conceptual breakthrough; once that had been established, what was now called for were some "quick and dirty" experiments to establish the validity of the proposition.[21] The task of carrying out these hypothesis-proving laboratory experiments fell to Ron Koenig, a Yale biochemistry graduate, who was in the first class of students in the fledgling Rockefeller/Cornell MD-PhD program. When starting out on a career in biomedical science, early exposure to an inspiring and diligent mentor can be defining; for Koenig, the quest to find just such an individual led him to Cerami's door. "I don't think I've ever met someone like him, he's unique. People [in the world outside] didn't know him then, but when I asked around at the Rockefeller, I was told, 'Oh, that guy is really going to make his mark on science....' But I was attracted by his youth, and because he was so excited about learning new things and so excited about science. It was obvious that he would care about working with me and not just ignore me."[22] Cerami is a scientist of rigorous principles and a demanding mentor, described as having a "hot presence in the lab,"[23] and as a young man, requiring little sleep, he pursued new challenges with a manic energy.[24] Cerami's management style was aimed at stimulating enthusiasm in researchers so that they would work around the clock and come up with new ideas for both him and themselves. But what Cerami did not know when he assigned the HbA1c study to Koenig as his PhD thesis project was that the young student was to prove "by far the most brilliant experimentalist that I've ever worked with."[25]

Working together, the first experiments were on mice to find out whether diabetic mice also had the mouse equivalent of human HbA1c. Applying the same method used for human blood, Koenig was able to show that diabetic mice had a minor hemoglobin fraction that corresponded to that seen with hemoglobin A1c in human red blood cells and that diabetic animals had 2.8 times more than nondiabetic mice. The red blood cell is exceptional in that all of the hemoglobin and other proteins in the cell are produced primarily when the cell resides in the bone marrow. The question was, When was HbA1c made?[26] In the process of contemplating this question, Koenig experienced a scientific revelation; his imagination guided him around formidable obstacles and in a completely unpredicted way. "That experiment was the first that I thought of myself. And when it happened, even though it was many years ago, I honestly remember being struck by the feeling *that I can't believe these ideas just came into my head. I don't know from where, or how, or if I'll have another one as long as I live. Because I don't know how these things happen.*"[27] Cerami always wanted to see data and pressed his researchers for primary results and hence the propensity to push for so-called quick-and-dirty experiments; although they might be easy to criticize methodologically, they would at least give an inkling if the path chosen was going in the right direction. However, Koenig's experiment was the embodiment of scientific sophistication and uncovered the mysteries of what was A1c and its biological significance. Contemplating these powerful questions, Koenig devised an ingenious strategy: "The idea was that we would radiolabel the hemoglobin in a normal mouse, later we transfused that, and split it into two portions; and transfused one half into a genetically diabetic mouse recipient that had high A1c, and the other half into a normal mouse that didn't have high A1c, then we could track the radioactivity in the A1c versus the normal hemoglobin over time, and this would tell us when HbA1c was made in the erythrocyte [red blood cell]."[28]

When it came to working in the lab, Cerami was uncompromising, dedicated, and single-minded, and in a similar fashion to Howard Florey, who pioneered the therapeutic discovery of penicillin, what he liked most "was the telling experiment."[29] But a fundamental worry for any inexperienced experimenter is safety. Accordingly, when Koenig was told by his boss to go ahead with the experiment "but don't contaminate the whole lab," he was understandably circumspect. "I was nervous because we had to inject a whole lot of radioactive iron into the tail veins of mice, which was not an easy thing to do. So I asked our lab technician, James Leong, who was incredibly good at these detailed things to inject the mice tails, as I didn't want to screw up and get into trouble. And I think Tony was initially skeptical about the value of the experiment, but when we saw the data, we were both excited."[30]

The researchers found that the rate of synthesis of A1c was linear throughout the life of the erythrocyte and that was made faster if that erythrocyte was living in a diabetic environment rather than in a normal mouse. It had nothing to do with the type of mouse that the blood or red cells came from; it had everything to do with the environment that the red blood cells were living in.[31] Tellingly, in this first article, they suggested that measurement of hemoglobin A1c would be related to metabolic control, and the reactive substance that reacted with hemoglobin could be responsible for the complications of diabetes. Because the adult red blood cell does not have a nucleus and does not synthesize protein, the production of HbA1c had to come about, Cerami reasoned, by a nonenzymatic reaction. The ability to theoretically understand a biological process before it is proved was one of Cerami's most important talents.

These breakthrough discoveries created genuine elation and gave Koenig the opportunity to see, at first hand, the clarity of Cerami's scientific instinct about the reactions that can happen between small molecules and biological systems that are not enzymatically catalyzed. "Tony sees things very quickly, and most other people, including myself, are not so good at seeing and making connections, thinking broadly. And when Tony would make some fundamental observation, you would say, 'That's obvious, why didn't I see that?' So that is the essence of Tony."[32]

Further work showed that the structure of HbA1c was an Amadori product of glucose attached to the amino terminus of hemoglobin,[33] and both Cerami and Koenig believed that the findings were potentially of clinical importance.[34] HbA1c is based on the principle that red blood cells live for 120 days. Every day, some blood cells are born while others die, and within the life cycle of a normal erythrocyte, 4.5 to 5 percent of its molecules bind to glucose. But, if the glucose is elevated for any significant period in a systematic way, then the measurement of HbA1c immediately picks up this increase. Also, it is worth remembering that the clinical status of diabetes was very much different in the 1970s than it is today. For example, endocrinologists did not regard it as an endocrine disease; it was seen as just another part of internal medicine.[35] Whereas today, the position has been entirely reversed, with diabetes being the most common endocrine disease diagnosed in the United States. Cerami's scientific imagination was untroubled by the large gaps in the physiological understanding of the disease; in fact, their existence only served to press him forward into the unknown. Koenig too recognized the value of disease-orientated research and the clinical deficiencies that he and Cerami had to contend with. "We both felt that what we were doing was potentially clinically important, but diabetes was in a totally different place back then. I wasn't convinced that it would be a useful every day clinical tool because a number of things were missing: the therapeutic tools were not equal to the task of glucose control, and also, no one had yet carried out a trial to prove the dangers of hypoglycemia. So my thinking was more like, 'this is going to be a cool research tool,' but whether it is actually going to be useful in management of diabetes is unknown because who knows where technology is going to go?"[36] At the time this work was being carried out, a febrile debate was taking place about whether the complications of diabetes were exacerbated by poor metabolic control. There were two schools of thought—the doctors who believed in "tight control" and those who did not believe that metabolic control was important and thus promoted "loose control."[37] This dichotomy offered the researchers an opportunity to provide some reliable evidence for the clinicians on both sides of the doctrinaire divide. "We arranged to obtain blood samples from two institutions," Cerami recalled, "representing each point of view. To our great surprise, the HbA1c values were between 11% and 13% from both institutions compared with values of 4–6% in non-diabetics."[38] Clearly, this implied that care of patients with diabetes was deficient and that clinical instinct, no matter how passionately pursued, was no substitute for evidence-based research.

One evening, over dinner in New York City, Cerami outlined his thinking on diabetes to Gerald Bernstein, a physician and endocrinologist. Bernstein had a special interest in metabolism and recalled that, when the conversation turned to hemoglobin molecules and glucose, "Tony said, 'my mother has diabetes—I wonder whether the amount of glucose on her hemoglobin is the same?'" To show that diabetic control as measured by glucose in the urine was related to HbA1c in the blood, the researchers, in collaboration with Joe Williamson, admitted diabetic patients into The Rockefeller University Hospital. Cerami's mother was immediately recruited into the study and lived at the hospital for over a year. Far from feeling alienated by her surrounding, Koenig remembered a wonderful, friendly woman. "She was our first patient, and it was a lot of fun having her around. I don't think Tony felt any extra anxiety; he believed that he was going to do his mother some good."[39] In fact, the hospital became the focal point of family life, with Cerami bringing in his two children, Ethan and Carla, to visit his mother on Saturday mornings. Over time, the patients were brought into good metabolic control, with the HbA1c values falling to values that were seen in normal patients.[40] Further studies in diabetic patients showed that HbA1c correlated with glucose control. What had started out as Cerami's hypothesis that HbA1c was a nonenzymatic reaction between glucose and hemoglobin became the salvation for his mother as her HbA1c levels came back to normal during her hospitalization and remained stable for several years.[41] By showing experimentally in both humans and animals that glucose became attached to one end of the beta chain running ahead of the hemoglobin, and that critical levels of sugar in the blood would be mirrored by the A1c level, a diagnostic advance was formed in understanding the mechanism of the disease.[42]

The success of the clinical study undertaken at The Rockefeller University Hospital and Cerami's daily visits there gave him the opportunity to discuss ideas with the remarkable physician-scientist Henry Kunkel. A laconic, thoughtful, and shy man, Kunkle was primarily dedicated to understanding immune dysfunction. Although the men were separated by age and discipline, Kunkle was Cerami's intellectual guiding light.[43] Kunkel defined the inherent autoimmune character of diseases such as rheumatoid arthritis; moreover, his concentration on disease-focused research and being able to delve deeply into the meaning and significance of an observation became the defining characteristics of Cerami's life in biomedical science. Many years later, Cerami wrote, "In my fantasies I frequently imagine being able to explain to Henry the concepts that we have developed since he died. He would have been interested and would have many astute questions of how to go forward."[44]

Early in his career, Cerami learned that science does not always win and that more critical than being right is being believed. Accordingly, the introduction of the HbA1c test to the medical community was met with skepticism when it was first introduced. For example, when Cerami suggested to the administrators of The Rockefeller University that they should patent his measurement of HbA1c as a method to measure metabolic control of diabetes, he was told that the idea was not financially viable and that several influential diabetologists did not think that the test would be of interest to their patients. In their defense, in the 1970s, widespread clinical testing was not feasible because it took a trained technician twenty-four hours to prepare patient samples, run them on a floor-to-ceiling ion exchange column and collect fractions in a fraction collector, and then read the tubes and calculate the data. In addition, the big controversy in the medical profession at the time was whether hyperglycemia had anything to do with diabetic complications or not. If not, then why measure HbA1c? Ultimately, the test was never patented, and this proved a salutary lesson; for the rest of his career, Cerami's disease-focused research produced scientific discoveries that were scrupulously protected by intellectual property patents. The recognition that his research work was motivated by a desire to promote patient care was never in doubt. Equally, it was widely recognized that Cerami was a translational scientist who operated on the business–biology frontier.[45]

One of the first groups of clinicians to embrace the concept of monitoring HbA1c was obstetricians who looked after pregnant patients with type 1 diabetes. At the time, the incidence of birth defects in children born to these mothers was over 20 percent. By promoting tight control of blood glucose through the use of HbA1c measurement, it was possible to reduce the incidence of birth defects to that found in nondiabetics.[46] Further vindication of the utility of glucose control came from the evidence of two large long-term studies of diabetic patients. The Diabetes Control and Complications Trial,[47] which was carried out by the National Institutes of Health from 1983 to 1993, showed that the onset and progression of diabetic complications of the eye and kidney were significantly reduced in patients with type 1 diabetes who had stricter glycemic control, as shown by HbA1c measurements. Just as compelling were the findings of the UK Prospective Diabetes Study Group[48] investigation of patients with type 2 diabetes that showed unequivocally the importance of glycemic control to reducing morbidity and mortality.

The HbA1c research was only the beginning of Cerami's lab's involvement in diabetes; soon attention was turned to the other complication of the disease and the complex chemical reactions of glucose with proteins in the body.[49] Cerami's work has been important to diabetologists because it alerted them to the damage that HbA1c was doing to the kidney.[50] In recognition of his elucidation of the biological complexities of the disease, in 1999, Cerami was awarded the Banting Medal of the American Diabetes Association. Gerald Bernstein, then president of the institution, acknowledges that it was incisive thinking and biochemical intuition that were the outstanding features of Cerami's translational philosophy. "Tony Cerami has the extraordinary capability of observing and then applying science to his observations, because nothing is an accident to him. Everything is thought out and then rigid science is applied. And I said if I'm going to give that award then

I need to look at somebody who has changed the base of everything—and that was Tony." Today, the HbA1c test has become the defining measurement for assessing diabetes management and is the Food and Drug Administration's benchmark for judging new diabetes drugs. During the first decade of the existence of the Laboratory of Medical Biochemistry, Cerami could often be found sitting in his subterranean office, looking out at an expanse of beautiful green ivy and thinking of the future. The foundations had been laid for a new research project that recognized that the reaction of glucose with proteins in the body could cause disease. This realization presented a fundamental human dilemma: that while glucose is essential for life, it is also a harbinger of aging and death.

6 · GLUCOSE, AGING, AND THE CROSS-LINKING OF BIOLOGY AND BUSINESS

Truth arises more readily from error than from confusion.

—Francis Bacon, *Novum Organum*, 1620

While progress in the understanding and cure of some diseases over the past seventy years has been impressive, other conditions remain stubbornly and tragically intractable. The immunologist Peter Medawar summed up the challenge as "the art of the soluble," suggesting that there seems to be a certain time when some biomedical questions are especially ripe for answering, whereas other problems remain elusive and out of reach.[1] When Cerami made the discovery that glucose, once considered biologically inert, could permanently alter some of the body's proteins, he realized that one of humanity's most enduring questions might be partially resolvable: was glucose in fact implicated in the human aging process?[2] The hypothesis formed a natural progression both scientifically and chemically from Cerami's pioneering work on A1c and in doing so opened up a completely new area of biological investigation. His innate interest in the impact of nonenzymatic chemistry led him to develop the theory that glucose and other reducing sugars could react with proteins and nucleic acids without the aid of enzymes to form a series of stable covalent adducts that permanently alter some proteins (drawing them together). These chemical linkages on A1c, nerve, lens, and kidney proteins—in exactly the same place in their amino acid sequence—could lead to toxicity and correspondingly contribute to age-associated declines in the functioning of cells and tissues.[3]

Cerami had arrived at this assumption based on his observation that the complications of aging occurred at a younger age in diabetics as a result of their higher blood glucose levels.[4] This accelerated form of aging leads diabetic patients to present with the age-related diseases of heart attack, stroke, cataract, atherosclerosis—a disorder of the artery wall—and kidney disease prematurely. The loss of biological function by the nonenzymatic reaction of glucose with proteins and nucleic acids offered a new way to explain the chemical basis of aging.[5] Cerami named the nature of this biological phenomenon "advanced glycosylation end products" (AGEs). It is important to remember that Cerami was not being biologically naive or narrow in his thinking: he recognized that other forms of aging could be occurring simultaneously. Free radical damage to proteins and DNA was self-evident (and indeed was an area of research that Cerami pioneered), but it was the slowly formed glucose-derived compounds that captivated his imagination. The early studies initiated in his lab convinced him, and his growing team of scientific disciples, that aging was linked to the process that takes place when food is cooked.[6] In advancing a new metabolic theory to explain diabetic complications, he set in motion a new area of investigation not only for his own laboratory but also for the wider biomedical world.

Before examining whether aging itself has any direct effects on the development of disease, it may be useful to consider whether there is any fundamental biological process that can usefully be labeled *aging*. This is exactly the question that the British epidemiologists Richard Doll and Richard Peto asked in their deliberately tendentious article "There Is No Such Thing as Aging."[7] The researchers inquired if aging could be defined as "baldness, greyness, dementia, wisdom, vascular disease, preneoplastic changes, immunological deterioration, collagen cross linking, or genetic changes in particular somatic cells?" Their article went on to suggest that what was really needed to advance the scientific study of aging was experimental hypotheses: "if we want to understand the mechanisms by which lung cancer arises we should study these and not the mechanisms of some other age related phenomenon such as the menopause; conversely, if we want to understand the timing of the menopause, of the progressive loss of tissue elasticity due to cross linking of collagen, or of senile cataracts we should study each of them directly."[8] Gaining a better understanding of the detailed structures and mechanisms of nature's catalysts was exactly what Cerami set out to do. His objective was to understand why we age and how humans might be able to live longer and healthier lives.

In seeking to explain the relationship between glucose and aging, Cerami was following in a great inquisitorial tradition, as aging and the quest to delay or avoid its inevitability have occupied the minds of humankind since the time of Methuselah, who, according to legend, lived to the age of 969. A far more contemporary figure was the brilliantly insightful Russian immunologist Elie Metchnikoff, who posed a tantalizing question in his 1907 book *The Prolongation of Life*, "What is the maximum age a human being can reach?"[9] It is worth recalling that it has only been in the past two centuries that there has been much of a change in the pattern of mortality. For example, an individual born at any time before the middle of the eighteenth century had less than a 50 percent chance of surviving long enough to produce any children.[10] But since the 1950s, in high-income countries, life expectancy has improved more than in the entire previous span of human history. As a consequence, to adapt the thinking of the British epidemiologist William Farr, how people live and how—of what causes and at what ages—they die are among the most important questions that can be considered.[11] Biological and physical anthropologists have concluded that there appears to be no built-in genetic construction that sets a fixed limit on life span. Yet different species have characteristic average life spans, which does suggest that longevity is determined by some biological mechanism. For Metchnikoff, the way forward to "curing" aging—he saw it as a disease—was by altering the composition of the gut flora, and so persuasive was his thinking that he singlehandedly launched a global craze for yogurt. Today Metchnikoff is seen, among other things, as the godfather of probiotics research, who over a century ago devised a gastronomic plan to harness the natural ambrosia of the trillions of microbes that inhabit the human digestive tract to enable him to live to the age of 150. He offered this physiological law of aging: "I'm almost inclined to derive a general rule: the longer the large intestine, the shorter the life."[12] Alas when he died at the age of seventy-one in 1916, he felt agony on his deathbed that his premature death would discredit his teachings.[13]

Cerami too was interested in food, food processing, nutrition, and the cellular receptors that elicit a variety of pathophysiological responses.[14] As humans, we eat plant carbohydrates and animal proteins and turn them into glucose, ATP (adenosine triphosphate, which transports chemical energy within cells for metabolism), and human proteins. These proteins are long chains of linked amino acids, folded into specific conformations, or shapes, that determine their ability to function within a cell, and thus their folding and unfolding are essential to the chemistry of life.[15] In many parts of the human body, such as the skin or blood cells, proteins are constantly being replaced. But in the basic structure of humans—bones and joints, for example—proteins are not replaced after their original fabrication. Critically, the proteins in the lens of the eye are formed before we are born and are never replaced and thus make a useful subject for the study of aging. As a consequence, the first investigations of Cerami's laboratory into aging were targeted at the potential role of glycosylation of lens crystallins in diabetic cataract formation.[16]

He was joined in this investigation by Carol Rouser, a young student on the MD/PhD program jointly run by Cornell Medical School and The Rockefeller University, both in New York. In 1978, Cerami had become the codirector of this pioneering program, which provided his laboratory with access to a reservoir of highly capable intellects eager to learn more about his approach of looking at biology from a chemist's point of view. The attraction of working with Cerami, for Rouser, was that "he thought a lot about the reactions between small molecules and biological systems that are not enzymatically catalyzed."[17] The hypothesis driving the study was that as the lens proteins turn over very slowly, they are likely to build up glucose adducts, which become a factor in diabetic cataract formation. The nonenzymatic glycosylation reaction of glucose with proteins begins when amino groups react with aldehyde glucose to form a Schiff base (a type of joined-up clustering). Once formed, the unstable Schiff base of glucose can undergo an Amadori rearrangement (an organic reaction, important in carbohydrate chemistry) to form a more stable product. As in the case of the Schiff base (named after Hugo Schiff), the amount of Amadori product formed is related to the glucose concentration. Shortly after beginning the study, the researchers noticed the accumulation of yellow and brown pigment in cataractous lenses, and this pigment turned out to be a product of glucose modification that had undergone a process known as the Maillard reaction. The eponymous process is a chemical reaction between amino acids and reducing sugars that gives browned food its distinctive, appetizing flavor. The reaction was first documented in 1912 by the French chemist Louis Camille Maillard, and his original work had inspired food chemists to investigate this flavor-producing response because of its importance in the cooking and storage of food products.[18] In addition to forming during cooking, the Maillard products can even form in freezing temperatures, and thus meat stored in a deep freezer will become tough as a result of protein cross-linking if stored for more than a year.

Although Maillard had suggested that this chemistry would be important in biology and medicine, Cerami could not find any studies demonstrating that this protein reformation occurred in living organisms. However, intuitively he felt that it was the impact of nonenzymatic chemistry on biological systems that was playing a role in both the complications of diabetes and aging. Cerami was a very enthusiastic researcher and in the lab; his management style, according to Carol Rouser, was conspicuously "laissez faire," believing that it was a good idea to give a postdoc a project and then "turn them loose."[19] He was also careful to acknowledge and support young researchers, as one of his inviolable aims was to bring on a new generation of basic and applied scientific investigators, and the most efficient way of achieving this objective was by the practical handing on of the skills of laboratory bench-craft. "Learning by doing" remained a guiding principle throughout Cerami's professional life, and fortuitously for him, Vincent Monnier, a Swiss postdoc with a degree in medicine and chemistry, had joined the diabetes research section of the laboratory in 1977.[20] Although Monnier was not to know it at the time, when his boss asked him to look for Maillard products in biological samples, the project presaged the focus of his forty-year research career: understanding aging in relation to type 2 diabetes. When Monnier examined the literature on the complications of diabetes, glucose, and the chemistry of glycation, he stumbled across the intriguing term *browning*. He became convinced that the phenomenon of browning was a progressive chemical reaction, which led him to postulate that glycation, the browning reaction, was an ongoing process in the human body and might help to explain the cross-linking of proteins that is responsible for the stiffness that occurs with the progression of age.

Cerami's indisputable commitment to new scientific ideas was indicative of the gung-ho atmosphere at the The Rockefeller University,[21] and of course being a relatively young and charismatic researcher, he related well to students and postdocs. He aimed to protect and mentor his team and to instill a sense of adventure. Nevertheless, everyone in Cerami's lab was conscious that it was a scientifically "hot place to be":[22] the hours were long, competition was tough, and success had to be earned. For his part, Vincent Monnier had been used to a more traditional, hierarchical scientific structure in Switzerland. What he found astounding was not only the level of integration between medicine and chemistry but also how the results from work at the bench were being promoted in dramatic ways. "Maybe every other month," Monnier reflects, "a television crew would be filming in the lab—and you would never have seen a television crew in a lab in Europe."[23] In addition to being an outstanding experimental innovator, Cerami had another virtue: he knew exactly what had to be done next, and he made sure that his team got it done. "He was very excited about the project," recalled Vincent Monnier four decades later, "and the great thing was that he allowed me to pursue it all by myself."[24]

Very soon their research showed that humans also "brown" and that this browning happens at 98.6 degrees Fahrenheit and takes place over a lifetime.[25] Work at The Rockefeller University established that when glucose interacts with proteins, they undergo reformations that form on their collagen, leading to impairment of protein function. Cerami and his team proved that when glucose reacts with a protein, it binds the molecules of the protein together, making them tougher and less flexible—just as in food that has been overcooked. This cross-linking of proteins creates a hardening of human connective tissue throughout the body and plays a primary role in both the complications of diabetes and aging. Within a decade of conceiving the hypothesis, Cerami had initiated and defined advanced glycation end products as a chemical process to describe organismal aging, while the term *AGEs* appealed to him as a nomenclature because it gave etymological validation to his belief that the process described the central mechanism responsible for aging. As Cerami accumulated greater understanding of the molecular pathway by which aging leads to impairment of protein function, he began to envisage ways in which this process could be slowed, stopped, or even reversed. He envisaged the use of a chemotherapeutic compound that would *break* the cross-linking AGE bonds and form a key defense against aging. He knew it would take years to achieve, but his flexibility and willingness to engage in biomedical research outside his field of expertise was a defining thread running through his career in translational medicine. Intrinsically, he believed that to be successful, you had to have a plan and that standing firm, free of vacillation, was the single most important factor in the ability to stay the course in science, along with the constant inner incantation: *Think....*

During these years, Cerami was bold in both his scientific and personal life, which were often intriguingly and complicatedly intertwined. His first child, Carla, was born in 1966, followed by a son, Ethan, four years later. His children gave him an immense sense of joy and were the center of his universe. Like many of his colleagues at The Rockefeller University, Cerami was conscious that science was an all-consuming profession and that it took a huge effort to switch off from the apotheoses and apocalypses of the lab to come home to his children at night. The temptation was always there to read another scientific paper or to continue working on a problem that was so close to being solved. There just did not seem to be enough hours in the day anymore, and in the early 1970s, the changing social mores of the time began to undermine the traditional adhesive bonds of love, marriage, and kinship to such a degree that contracts entered into just a decade previously seemed to originate in another age entirely. New York City was at the center of this destabilizing societal vortex, and after more than a decade together, both Tony and Kathy became aware that they no longer moved at the same speed. There was little conscious serenity, and the feeling was that their marriage was slowly disintegrating.

This fragile situation was not helped when Cerami left New York to attend a conference on pharmacology being held in Greece in the summer of 1974. The symposium took place aboard an armada of vessels that traveled through the southern Aegean Sea, stopping along the way to visit Crete, Santorini, and other islands in The Cyclades. At the conference, Cerami met a young Greek medical student, Helen "Nellie" Vlassara. They fell in love, and so strong was the emotion that Cerami was determined to bring Helen back to New York City to live and work with him. But he was now confronted with a true moral dilemma: torn between the parental commitment to his children's happiness and well-being and the emotional lightness he now felt in Helen's company. In the event, it was decided that the children should remain with their mother in the family home and that Cerami should move to a large one-bedroom apartment in one of The Rockefeller University's dormitories. This enabled him to be with his children at the weekends and during vacations, but the situation was not helped when his mother also came to live him in the dormitory apartment! At weekends, it was a tight squeeze, and for quite some time, his family was in effect "camping" in the apartment and enjoying all of its chaotic claustrophobic fun.

In what turned out to be a dramatic episode, Cerami almost failed in his attempt to get Helen to the United States because of the chaos that followed the fall of the Greek military dictatorship in the summer of 1974. Between 1967 and 1974, Greece was governed by the Regime of the Colonels, a neofascist government so violent and harsh that then British Prime Minister Harold Wilson referred to it as a "bestial regime." Paralleling its brutality, the junta was morally puritanical and socially anachronistic. From the outset, the regime wanted to stem the tide of what it perceived as the left-wing decadence that was undermining civil society. As a consequence, the dictatorship banned mini-skirts for women and long hair for men, and great works of literature were also proscribed, including books by Shakespeare, Chekhov, and even Aristophanes. Unfortunately for Cerami and Helen, as they were making their way to the airport in Athens, the Turkish army's invasion of the island of Cyprus precipitated the fall of the dictatorship on July 24, 1974. A great national outpouring of suppressed emotion followed, power fell into the streets, and confusion reigned throughout the institutions of the state. This was the political maelstrom from which Helen and Cerami somehow were eventually able to extract themselves. They flew to New York unmolested by the dissolving forces of the dictatorship, but it had been a close call. This was not the only time that Cerami was caught up in dangerous political situations. In 1979, while on vacation on the island of St. Lucia with Ethan and Carla, he only avoided a hazardous confrontation between opposing political demonstrators by taking evasive action. On the evening of July 18, 1979, Cerami and his family were driving back to their hotel when a political rally of 4,000 people turned violent—rocks and bags of excrement where being thrown, and the stench of tear gas was in the air. Sensing the danger, and seeing that a makeshift roadblock was preventing them returning to their hotel, Cerami drove his children across rutted fields to safety. The unrest led to the burning down of the island's prison, and the authorities briefly lost control.[26]

Over much of the following three decades, as well as being bound together in marriage, Cerami and Helen were also scientific collaborators forming the nucleus of the team conducting research into AGEs in Cerami's lab. Together with her colleagues, Vlassara showed that AGEs were linked to a wide range of serious conditions, including vascular disease, kidney disease, obesity, Alzheimer's disease, and other so-called diseases of aging.[27] Additionally, Vlassara, building on the work of Maillard and other food chemists, suggested that it was possible to reduce the harmful effects of AGEs on the body as most of these compounds enter the body through the food that people eat.[28] This was a process of infusing modern meaning into a health concept communicated by Hippocrates: good health could be achieved though diet. Vlassara's work went on to show that the overconsumption of highly brown food, such as red meat, has a number of detrimental biological effects, while conversely, a diet that is less brown is generally going to be less palatable, leading to less food being consumed and a healthier body mass index.[29] According to Vlassara, "beef tends to have the highest levels of AGEs, followed by poultry and pork. Fish has more moderate AGE levels, while eggs and legumes . . . rank lowest on the AGE scale for proteins."[30] It had not escaped the notice of Vlassara and her coworkers that a possible panacea to the obesity epidemic in the United States was the promotion of the AGE-less gastronomy.[31] Moreover, it appeared that it was never too late to start a low-AGE diet,[32] and accordingly, Helen Vlassara wrote cookery books with recipes that signposted the way to eat food that was less biologically damaging. Amusingly, in one of those gentle touches of familial irony, Carla Cerami thought that Nellie's foray into the flourishing culinary publishing sector was somewhat incongruous, given that "Nellie probably wasn't the best cook in the family."[33] During the early years of the reconfigured Cerami family life, there may have been awkward moments of personality dynamics, but evidently Helen's grace and stability allowed her to calmly absorb the dramas that swirled around. Indeed, Nellie's presence was such a strong influence that she inspired Carla to study medicine and to take up the life of a translational scientist too.[34]

Creatively, the 1980s marked a prodigious period in Cerami's scientific life, and as the field of inquiry expanded, so too did the size and composition of his laboratory.[35] On Monday mornings, he would have freshly cut flowers arranged outside the door of his laboratory office. This stylish flourish, helping to make everything "just so,"[36] may have been afforded by the extra cash he had accumulated after giving up smoking the slim panatela cigars that he had become addicted to in his twenties. But one habit he was never able to shake was regularly walking through the lab to ask inquisitorially of each member of his team, "What's new?" Some of the more experienced researchers held something noteworthy in reserve for just such an occasion,[37] but with the lab's field of research being so wide, incorporating AGEs, the cytokine theory of disease, and parasitology, the reply was invariably *a lot*. There was a sense of a gathering momentum, and the earlier work treating sickle cell disease had gained the lab favorable publicity that Cerami greatly enjoyed,[38] while there was also a more general recognition that his researchers were explorers seeking insights at the frontiers of science. Cerami's objective was to encourage his team to think broadly about solutions, to find new ways to understand and treat disease, and then to materially support their efforts as best he could.

During these years of high-yield science, Cerami was frequently in and out of the lab, looking for new revenue streams to finance his expanding research program. Like many of his contemporaries, he wrote successful National Institutes of Health (NIH) grant applications, but with funding for translational medicine notoriously scarce, he increasingly managed his large laboratory more in the style of a businessman-entrepreneur than along the lines of a traditional Rockefeller scientist.[39] Being an outlier for the more commercially minded academic scientist suited Cerami and fused succinctly with The Rockefeller University's new strategy of encouraging faculty to work one day a week on non-Rockefeller business in the private or nonprofit sectors of their related fields.[40] Because of his celebrated contributions to understanding aging and seeking ways to allow people to live longer and healthier lives, in 1983, Cerami was approached by the Brookdale Foundation, a charity dedicated to enhancing the quality of life of America's elderly. Headquartered in his native New Jersey, the foundation invited Cerami to become its senior scientific fellow and a member of its advisory board. The new opportunity offered generous support for his work on aging[41] and gave occasion to meet the inspirational psychiatrist, Robert Butler, who also served on the foundation's advisory board. The two men shared the common goal of altering society's perceptions of aging and the aged. Indeed, "Bob" Butler was a charismatic and persuasive scientist-gerontologist who, through his persistence in support of older people, was perhaps the key factor in transforming geriatrics into a full discipline of medicine.[42] A pioneering old age psychiatrist, Butler helped to found the National Institute on Aging (NIA) and served as its first director before leaving in 1982 to become founding chairman of the department of geriatrics and adult development at Mount Sinai School of Medicine, New York—the first geriatrics department in the United States.[43] Famously in the late 1960s, Butler, having appropriated a linguistic classification from the terms *sexism* and *racism*, introduced the noun *ageism* into the lexicon, to describe the stigma faced by older people in American society. Cerami's admiration for Butler's evangelism concentrated his mind anew to find novel biomedical ways to reduce the unnecessary pain and suffering of aging.

At the same time that Cerami was framing a strategy to finance an innovative translational medicine program, the AGE section of his lab welcomed a new member, Michael Brownlee. The focus of Brownlee's work before, during, and after his eight years working with Cerami at The Rockefeller University was understanding the pathogenesis of diabetic complications and the development of potential therapies to prevent or arrest their progression. Aligned to a profound interest in the natural history of the disease, Brownlee had a personal stake in contributing to the science of diabetology as he himself had type 1 diabetes. The realities of the social and physiological ramifications of the disease were brought home to Brownlee when he attended an interview at Duke University Medical School. In a casual, almost matter-of-fact way, the interviewer outlined the dystopian prognosis of Brownlee's condition and asked, "Why should you be taught medicine here? You've got type 1 diabetes and you will be dead before your mid-thirties while someone else could take that place and treat patients until they are in their seventies."[44] Happily, Brownlee found an established professor at Duke with type 1 diabetes who kindly wrote the young student a letter of support, and he was duly accepted into the medical school.

The newly constituted AGE team made impressive progress by applying the biochemical discoveries previously made at The Rockefeller University by Stanford Moore,[45] who had developed the first automated amino acid analyzer that enabled the determination of protein sequences.[46] Moore's work described the connection between the chemical structure and catalytic activity of the ribonuclease molecule; this discovery was critical in understanding how a biological malfunction might be repaired in the human body. Moore's thinking was of great theoretical importance to Cerami's team, and throughout the 1980s, they attempted to pharmacologically intervene with AGE formation or AGE cross-linking.[47] The catalyst for their most audacious scientific undertaking was a paper that advanced a theory on diabetic vascular disease that had caught the attention of Michael Brownlee.[48] "The hypothesis," Brownlee remembers, "was that the increased concentrations of histamine played a central role, and in one these papers the scientists used a compound to inhibit the enzyme that synthesizes histamine from the amino acid, whereas I thought that the beneficial effect they saw was in fact due to the inhibition of AGE formation by a hydrazine part of the compound."[49] Brownlee felt compelled to find a way to put his interpretation of the biological evidence to the test. But any attempt to pharmacologically intervene to prevent the Amadori product from cross-linking with other proteins via their amino groups would require the insights of a brilliant organic chemist. Peter Ulrich, another member of Cerami's lab, fitted the bill perfectly, and off the top of his head, he recited to Brownlee a list of potential candidates that would elevate levels of histamine rather than reduce them. The first molecule he cited, aminoguanidine, had an amino group attached to positively charged guanidine, which is always charged at neutral pH. This inhibits the free amino group from becoming protonated, forming a bond, and thus allows it to be readily able to react with carbonyl groups.[50] Cerami's team immediately sought verifiable, evidence-based results of the effectiveness of aminoguanidine: in laboratory tests on rats, the drug did prevent random cross-linking of proteins such as collagen in blood vessels. The findings were published in *Science* and suggested that aminoguanidine could prove useful in reducing the blood vessel stiffening that is one of the most damaging effects of aging.[51] The researchers suggested a potential clinical role for aminoguanidine in the future treatment of chronic diabetic complications. Emboldened by the findings, Cerami told the *New York Times* that "the experimental drug was the first ever found to prevent the damaging cross-linking" of proteins.[52] With an estimated 11 million diabetics in the United States at the time, the AGE team believed that aminoguanidine's potential ability to prevent arteriosclerosis (reduced arterial elasticity) and aging in diabetics offered "an exciting clinical possibility that needs further investigation."[53]

With the likelihood of having discovered such a promising cross-linking inhibitor therapeutic, the AGE team decided that they should patent their invention. Cerami had learned a valuable lesson from the failure of The Rockefeller University to patent his HbA1c diagnostic test even though he had offered to personally pay for the patenting fees. But this offer had been rejected[54] by the financially conservative university, which had little experience of commercializing the scientific discoveries made in its laboratories. Cerami now believes that had The Rockefeller University patented the test that was subsequently used across the world to diagnose and manage diabetes, licensing fees would have supported numerous research programs, while the patent itself would have elevated his own standing in the highly competitive world of academic science and brought some much needed extra money at a time when he was going through a painful divorce. Philosophically, Cerami was also heartfelt in his belief in intellectual property (IP) as a fundamental building block in how scientists contribute to the growth of scientific knowledge. This view of protecting the creations of scientific intellects contradicted that of Sir John Sulston, the British biologist best known for his pioneering work on the human genome who celebrated the ideals of open access and challenged on ethical and scientific grounds a model in which access to data would be controlled by commercial license agreements.[55] Cerami also clearly recognized that without a sense of cooperation and open communication resultant from unfettered collaboration, science becomes a closed culture—nevertheless, he was adamant in the belief that it was part of his scientific doctrine "to go to court to protect your work."[56] Accordingly, the patent process went ahead, with Brownlee listed as the senior inventor, Cerami as first inventor, and Peter Ulrich as the second inventor.

If Cerami's earlier attempts to inject an element of entrepreneurialism at The Rockefeller University had been given a frosty reception, the situation was rapidly changing. The ecosystem of academic scientists and institutions being involved in commercial enterprises was only in its infancy, but by the middle of the 1980s, a new economic template was emerging. The breakthrough company in this collaboration between venture capitalism and biochemistry was Genentech, established in 1976 and highly successful in raising large amounts of capital.[57] Genentech was the first modern biotechnology company, and it was responsible for producing the first recombinant DNA drug, human insulin, named Humulin, launched in 1982.[58] In addition, academic institutions were slowly reevaluating the potentially lucrative biotechnology field as a result of the vast sums of money provided to Columbia University from a family of patents known as the "Axel patents," which were issued in 1983. Richard Axel was a molecular biologist at Columbia University who was awarded the Nobel Prize in Physiology or Medicine in 2004. The eponymous patents covered the technique of cotransformation via transfection, a process that enabled foreign DNA to be inserted into a host cell to produce certain proteins. This technique was widely taken up by pharmaceutical companies to make, among other things, recombinant insulin and recombinant growth hormone. These patents, by making Columbia the recipient of hundreds of millions of dollars, had the effect of changing the culture within academic institutions: where once there was reluctance, now there was enthusiasm given the obvious boost to university coffers that internally produced patentable discoveries could provide.

In fact, the climate was such that some were beginning to have unrealistic expectations about biotechnology and its place in medicine's armamentarium. This was the heady atmosphere that framed the high-yield, translational work of Cerami's lab: his disease-focused research was not only scientifically exciting, offering as it did the possibility of predicting an outcome before it is observed in a clinical setting, but tellingly, it also resonated with the financial and institutional values of the time. For his part, Cerami was determined to capitalize on the growing presence of the ethics of the market in some areas of public-funded—NIH—academic science. Following negotiations with the lawyer for The Rockefeller University, William H. Griesar, Cerami established the biotechnology startup company Geritech in 1986, founded on the technologies developed by him and his team. The etymology of the company's name alluded to Cerami's general theory of aging,[59] the complications associated with diabetes, a recognition of the changing demography of the U.S. population, and also the influence of Bob Butler. The firm went on to form a strategic alliance with the Japanese drug company Yamanouchi Pharmaceuticals in 1989. The two firms joined forces to collaborate on the research, development, and commercialization of Geritech's diabetes drugs. In return, Geritech received a substantial payment.[60] Almost immediately, however, in preparation for the company to go public and be traded on the stock market, it was decided on the advice of a brand-naming agency that a catchier name was required, and subsequently, Geritech became transmogrified into Alteon—*alt* means *old* in German—with offices in Ramsey, New Jersey. Cerami took a seat on the board, received research funding from the company, and, together with Michael Brownlee, sat on the startup's scientific board. Initial funding was provided by a medically trained venture capitalist, Richard Proper, who had offices in the TransAmerica Pyramid Building in San Francisco. In 1990, Alteon formed an alliance with Marion Merrell Dow, a $2.4 billion pharmaceutical division of the Dow Chemical Company. The objective of the partnership was to collaborate on the development, commercialization, and marketing of Alteon's diabetes and antiaging products. At the time of the arrangement, phase I trials on aminoguanidine had been completed, but phase II and phase III trials were just about to begin. And as Tony Cerami knew only too well, the biggest challenge in translational medicine was making the move from animal trials to trials in patients. The question of the hour was, Could sclerotic stiffness be prevented and reversed in humans?

This combination of febrile activity and the relentless added weight of expectations from commercial partners took its toll on Cerami and had a destabilizing effect on the emotional dynamics coursing through his lab. Exceptional individuals have strong opinions, views, and a relentless drive, but the best ones are also sensitive. First and most important, how can scientists be motivated, controlled, and guided to conjure up new ideas? Managing and inspiring them can be both confusing and complex, as scientists (like many of us) can be wayward, stubborn, volatile, and egotistic. Learning how to embrace high-maintenance colleagues who are also competitors can be an essential quality. Sometimes, laboratory science requires a benevolent dictator: someone kind but strong or, conversely, an individual who by the sheer brilliance of their intellect and indomitable presence is able to mold a scientific team into a collective greater than could have been imagined. One such archetype was Howard Florey, the resolute Australian pathologist. Florey was not particularly warm or charismatic in the conventional meaning of the word. It seems, for instance, that he was a man incapable of giving praise, and on occasion, he would greet people in the corridors of his fiefdom, the William Dunn School—where Cerami once contemplated working—with the heartless greeting, "Still going backwards?" Deflationary comments were his stock-in-trade, and almost universally, he used surnames in addressing or talking about people, an adherence to formal modes of address that was a mechanism by which Florey kept familiarity at bay.[61] Conversely, Cerami's personality was very different: he was warm, friendly, approachable, and, in addition, charming. As Albert Camus put it in The Fall, charm is a way of getting people to say yes before you have told them what you want. The relationship was of course reciprocated; it is important to recognize the vital role of personality in driving science and the scientific process. It was widely recognized that Cerami loved working with young people in the lab and had the enviable ability to find, in a very artistic way, a means of mentoring that drove or inspired young people in a manner that they wanted to be developed or develop themselves.[62] But there were chinks in Cerami's armor. Periodically, it was felt by some that he considered people in very black-and-white terms, finding it difficult to understand that there were shades of gray; he could also be emotionally sensitive, and relationships that had been established over many years deteriorated into extended periods of what in the lab became known as "the silent treatment," and on occasion, this led to something closer to excommunication.

Nevertheless, leading a large laboratory at a time when the efficacy of aminoguanidine in diabetic patients was about to be determined by a randomized controlled trial (RCT) proved extremely challenging. Vincent Monnier, who witnessed some of the personal and scientific schisms that occurred during this period, recognized the leitmotifs of bridge building and bridge burning as concurrent narratives in Cerami's life in science. Inherently, he admired how his boss could cope with the enormous pressures that occupy the mind of those responsible for transforming speculative experiments into research programs while at the same time propelling forward the careers of ambitious scientists.[63] Undoubtedly for Cerami, further anxiety also came in the form of the shadowy, ever-present fear that permeates the minds of scientists: the dread of being preempted. Inexorably, the 1980s and 1990s was a period of intense and growing competition for Cerami's lab, with well-funded groups from Harvard and other institutions snapping at their heels, which in turn fostered a sense of unease that was not always healthy and may have contributed to oscillations in temperament.

What is certain, however, is that while in terms of their respective personalities, styles of personnel management, and scientific focus, Tony Cerami and Howard Florey shared little in common, on one subject there was unanimity: what they both liked most was the simple effective experiment. "Ideas are cheap," Cerami would opine, "it's experiments that are important to understand." Yet unlike Florey's work on penicillin, where the impact was so profound that no RCT was needed to prove its efficacy, Cerami inhabited a different era with more stringent and complex evaluations. In the modern world, RCTs introduced by the U.K. Medical Research Council in the 1940s have become the essential scientific arbiter—or otherwise—through which drugs, treatments, or other interventions are translated from the laboratory to the clinic.[64] For Cerami and his colleagues, their AGE drug aminoguanidine was going to be tested for safety and effectiveness by the methods that underpin the RCT: the basic principles of randomization, replication, and unbiased observation. The results of the trial were to be portentous.

The clinical trial (ACTION 1) in patients with type 1 diabetes and end-stage renal disease was performed over two to four years.[65] Although there were positive clinical effects observed in patients receiving the drug—aminoguanidine had been rebranded "Pimagedine" by Alteon—the treatment groups did not reach statistical significance[66] over the placebo group for the primary end point of a doubling of serum creatinine.[67] Therefore, as an effective therapy, the drug was a failure. Despite failing to cross the line of clinical viability, the ACTION 1 randomized, double-masked, placebo-controlled study in 690 patients was far from damning. While the experiment "did not demonstrate a statistically significant beneficial effect of pimagedine on the progression of overt nephropathy resulting from type 1 diabetes, it [was] noteworthy in providing the first clinical proof of the concept that inhibiting advanced glycation end product formation can result in a clinically important attenuation of the serious complications of type 1 diabetes mellitus."[68] In mitigation, neuropathy, the numbness or weakness of nerves in toes, fingers, hands, and feet, can be difficult to quantify, and on the plus side, the drug was neither dangerous nor unsuccessful. In fact, it did show a decrease in some of the most damaging aspects of the disease. For his part, Cerami felt that the Food and Drug

Administration (FDA) had demanded unrealistic end-point parameters for the demonstration of safety and advocacy, and he petitioned them on several occasions. His appeals did not fall entirely on deaf ears, with some members of the FDA being understanding and helpful, but in this instance, Cerami failed to persuade the FDA to approve the molecule for clinical use.[69] More damaging news came in March 1998, when Alteon announced that it had been advised that it should discontinue its phase III trial of pimagedine in non-insulin-dependent type 2 diabetes patients with overt nephropathy after the trial's external safety monitoring committee found an increased risk of side effects in the treatment group. The die was cast, and to Cerami's disappointment, the development of the compound was halted.[70]

Cerami learned much from the failures of these translational studies, not least that the selection of clear objective end points that can quickly identify efficacy is of paramount importance. This became a vital element in the clinical development strategies for all the compounds on which he subsequently worked, as did the desire to encourage a new generation of translational scientists to discover new drugs to treat diabetic patients who develop retinopathy, neuropathy, and cardiovascular disease.[71] Indeed, it should not be forgotten that the identification of AGEs not only established a completely new field of scientific research but also launched the stellar careers of a generation of physician-scientists whose work improved the lives of diabetic patients.

Although the compounds developed by the for-profit company Alteon failed to be translated into clinical use, it nevertheless constituted a very successful scientific startup that made The Rockefeller University many millions of dollars from their involvement.[72] On December 23, 1996, Cerami wrote to William Griesar, vice president and general counsel of The Rockefeller University, about the distribution of monies accruing to him and ten other members of his staff. "I am enclosing the names, addresses and percentages agreed to by the inventors of the AGE technology that was part of The Rockefeller University patent estate, that was licensed to Aleton Inc. in exchange for 672,000 shares of Alteon stock. As we discussed, at the time that The Rockefeller University sold stock on the open market, the inventors are entitled to share 50% of the first $100,000 and 10% of the income thereafter." Three weeks later, in a letter dated January 13, 1997, Griesar addressed Cerami's financial concerns. "The enclosed check represents your agreed percentage of the inventors' share of cash consideration received by the University for license rights granted to Alteon Inc. The University originally was given Alteon stock for the license rights and was restricted from selling it for some period. That stock has now been sold, however, and the inventors' share of the cash realized on such sales amounts to $884,457, to be divided among the inventors as they agree." Griesar's letter ended with a paragraph of unrestrained praise for Cerami: "Your scientific efforts at the University have been extraordinary and, in this instance, have yielded significant financial reward both for the university and for you individually (33.0556%). With this check comes my thanks, on behalf of the entire University community, for your fine work."

Indeed, Alteon Inc. remained a lucrative financial lifeline for Cerami, paying him annual consultation fees of $250,000 in 1998. This intimate relationship with pharmaceutical companies, cross-linking as it did the worlds of biology and business, led him in a moment of introspection to feel that his status had become blurred by association: "People don't understand who I am. The academics might think I'm a business guy, seeing me as someone making money. I was also criticized because I'm not medically qualified, not a specialist—which is true."[73] Resentment and ridicule aside, throughout those years at the end of the twentieth century, he never lost sight of why he made his life in medical research—to gain useful knowledge and understand why a disease happened. Cerami has always been conscious of the constant tensions that exist in his life scientific that transcend categories and norms: the struggle between money and science, between position and opposition that have driven him inexorably forward on a trajectory guided by a complex mixture of curiosity, ego, brilliance, a fear of boredom, and the excitement of the new. The objectives were the prevention, treatment, and understanding of disease, and all three were well worth pursuing.

Just as Cerami has been undeterred, perhaps even bolstered by failure, for investigators pursuing basic science in the hope of improving human health and longevity, Cerami's audacious attitude is the crystallization of discovery science at its best: the process of identifying the new, the unknown, and the unexpected.[74] Following in the experimental slipstream of his two nineteenth-century scientific champions, Louis Pasteur and Paul Ehrlich, Cerami had succeeded in expanding the discipline of medical science, and in working with AGEs and diabetic-related diseases, he had also widened the parameters of the study of metabolic aging and encouraged others to enter the field.

7 · THE CONCEPTUAL BREAKTHROUGH

For a scientist, it is a unique experience to live through a period in which his field of endeavor comes to bloom…to listen to the sound of darkness crumbling.

—George Palade (in M. Farquhar, *George E. Palade 1912–2008*)

One autumn day in 1977, the dean of students at The Rockefeller University, biologist Jim Hirsch, arranged a lunch meeting to introduce his friend Kenneth S. Warren to Tony Cerami. Hirsh thought that Cerami might use the opportunity to subtly sound Warren out about funding the Laboratory of Medical Biochemistry's fledgling work in parasitology.[1] Earlier that year, John Knowles, president of the Rockefeller Foundation (RF), had appointed Warren to the post of director of health sciences at the foundation. Thus began Warren's career as a grant maker. From what in today's terms was a rather modest power base,[2] Warren helped to resurrect the RF's standing in international health after several decades' absence and established "one of the greatest initiatives in tropical medicine research that the world has witnessed."[3] Warren was hyperthymic; overflowing with energy and enthusiasm, the constants were a big smile and huge spectacles. He was a man of average height, but that was the only average thing about him. Ken Warren was a proselytizing parasitologist who wanted to use biomedical science to change the world. Warren believed that modern biological science was not being applied to infectious tropical diseases affecting some of the world's poorest people in Africa, Asia, and Latin America, and that change would only occur if basic science in clinical departments and medical schools became involved. He perfected the model in his own laboratory at Case Western Reserve University (Cleveland, Ohio) and had established his status as a renowned investigator of schistosomiasis.[4]

Warren's vision was to bring cost-effective health care to some of the poorest people in the global south, and his outstanding ability was his use of metrics to articulate health as an investment, not simply as expenditure. Furthermore, in the language of modern philanthropy, Warren had "convening power," which he used to mobilize powerful people, agencies, and institutions on behalf of the poor and the sick. It was this audacious ambition, to establish a network of laboratories that would apply the new biology of molecular medicine, immunology, epidemiology, and biochemistry to the parasitic diseases ubiquitous in tropical countries, that led Warren to Cerami's Laboratory of Medical Biochemistry. Immediately upon meeting, the scientists established that they shared a common interest: understanding the causes of disease and using that knowledge to alleviate suffering. Over lunch, they developed a genuine rapport based on a shared worldview that medical science was an important force for social change, and the meeting marked the beginning of a close personal friendship that only came to an end when Warren died of metastatic melanoma in 1996 at the age of sixty-seven.[5]

One of Warren's great achievements during his decade at the RF was the founding of the Great Neglected Diseases of Mankind Network (GND). There is no doubt that this program had a very important effect on the evolution of research on many neglected diseases, particularly those in the tropical belt.[6] The ambitious plan was to design a scientific program that would create "a network of high-quality investigators who would constitute a critical mass in this field, attract the brightest students and conduct research of excellence."[7] Of course, there was no selection committee or peer-review process involved, and the imperious-minded Warren personally chose the laboratories to be funded and persuaded some of the world's leading scientists to join, even though many had not previously worked on any neglected disease. Through sheer force of personality, using his inherent strengths as catalyzer, agitator, and matchmaker, Warren fused the network into a strike force that has left a profound legacy on global health thinking. Legendary names such as David Weatherall, Michael Sela, Hans Wigzell, and Gus Nossal were soon brought into Warren's privileged *family*, and others like Adel Mahmoud and John David became world famous through the GND.[8] The teams were to be multidisciplinary, and all members were to attend an annual meeting, which was crafted as a major social-scientific event. Moreover, the program affirmed one of Warren's sacrosanct beliefs, "that a significant part of the investigator's efforts would be spent in applied collaborative research with colleagues in developing countries."[9] In this sense, the project would establish global networks that would link what Warren termed "the bench to the bush, and the bush to the bench."[10] Over their historic lunch, which turned out to be a "smashing success,"[11] Warren, a communicator of beguiling intensity, outlined his vision for investigator-initiated approaches to disease control in the tropics. Few could fail to be persuaded by Warren's heartfelt, realistically costed advocacy; indeed, Cerami was not only impressed with the remarkable offer of $100,000 research funding every year for a decade, but equally "the dedication of Ken to the field of parasitology and the poor people of the world is an aspect of the GND that I will never forget."[12] The Warren-designed, RF-funded GND program marked a significant moment in the history of infectious diseases as it represented the first attempt by a big philanthropic organization to take on the global health agenda. It sought to get a new generation of the most talented scientists from across the globe to work on a defined list of parasitic diseases. For the geneticist John Bell, the importance of the GND was defined in its daring and

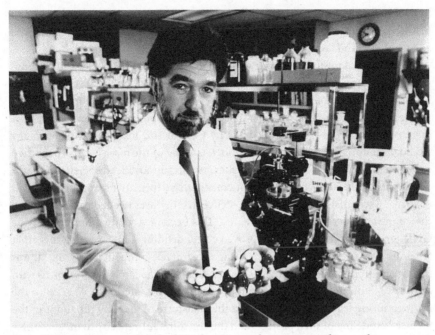

Cerami in his Laboratory of Medical Biochemistry—always interested in puzzles.

simple message: "here is the long-term funding, and these are the diseases that are causing the greatest burden of death and debility—now get after them."[13]

Research was at the heart of the GND. Warren's philosophy was to develop the science, line it up with the clinical problems, and move between the laboratory and the clinic—the clinic, in the case of the GND, being low-income countries in the tropics. This was translational medicine in a developing world setting: the long road back and forth between the bedside, the laboratory, and the community. The main focus of each GND unit continued to be an examination of the mechanisms of disease (i.e., finding out how things worked). The innovative nature of the program and why it synergized so perfectly with Cerami's scientific philosophy of using science to interact with the disease process was the concept of applying biochemical translational knowledge to the problems of parasitism, aligned to a belief that without fundamental investigations of the biology of these organisms, it would be very difficult to make progress in finding ways to control infection. The great neglected diseases were described by Warren as *great* in terms of prevalence and *neglected* in terms of the involvement of major international scientists and financial support. GND funding thus played a crucial role in expanding the horizons of parasitology by supporting a group of new researchers who reinvigorated the status of tropical medicine in the United States and beyond. A brilliant cohort of scientists who were spread across the world—including Zilton Andrade, Peter Perlmann, Dick Guerrant, Graham Mitchell, and Emanuela Handman—was supported by Warren and the RF to work on tropical diseases at a time when flexible long-term funding was rare and difficult to secure. In turn, all of these investigators have made a lasting contribution to disease control and human health, both as part of the GND program and in subsequent years.[14]

There is no doubt the Warren was a highly complex, eccentric, and at times polarizing figure, but these characteristics were tempered by the recognition that he was the architect of a great humanitarian vision.[15] He was also a brilliantly prophetic clinical scientist, and during that historic first lunch together in 1977, Warren stressed that the discoveries made by Cerami and his team in parasitology would undoubtedly lead to a greater understanding of the diseases that were then common in the United States and other economically advanced societies. Clearly, one significant reason why the network made such a formative impact on the lives of so many scientists was Warren's insistence that diseases needed to be studied in the countries where they were endemic. This became a vital component of the GND program, and for Cerami, it proved career defining. Little wonder, then, that ten years after their introductory meeting, Cerami felt compelled to write, "It was the most important lunch of my life, since it launched me into new unknowns with a group of dedicated people that I am proud to be associated with."[16] Perhaps the most enduring legacy can be found in the transformations brought about in the financial modeling of such projects and the concomitant capacity to incubate new talent and collaborative work. The actuarial model of Warren's RF program achieved remarkable results with only modest resources. During the eight-year period of its funded existence, the project involved 161 scientists and clinicians and 360 trainees, of whom 150 were from low-income countries, and resulted in the publication of 1,800 papers. This was all accomplished at the cost of approximately $15 million—a good rate of return by any standards.[17]

One member of that devoted team was his MD/PhD student Steven Meshnick, who had already begun to foster links with researchers from the global south—including Onesmo ole-MoiYoi at the International Laboratory for Research on Animal Diseases—along the lines that Warren had envisioned.[18] "I suppose," Meshnick later observed, "that it was me who got Tony interested in parasitology."[19] At the time, Cerami wanted to study malaria because he was attracted to high-risk projects that were difficult to fund,[20] but Meshnick had become captivated by trypanosomes, and so it was trypanosomes—specifically *Trypanosoma brucei*—that became their parasite of choice. Trypanosomes, organisms carried by the tsetse fly, cause three major diseases in humans—Chagas disease, leishmaniosis, and African trypanosomiasis (sleeping sickness)—and severe catabolic wasting and death in cattle. Collectively, both men set out to develop new drugs for African trypanosomiasis[21] and other orphan tropical diseases using Cerami's concept of rational drug design. Cerami had jettisoned the traditional empirical model of trial-and-error drug discovery—the empirical model—believing that the available treatments for human tropical diseases caused by parasitic trypanosomes lagged far behind the enormous advances in chemotherapy of bacterial diseases.[22] His modus operandi was to seek a better understanding of basic biochemistry and cell biology to determine how the metabolism of a parasite differed from the host's metabolism, to find an "Achilles' heel"[23] and to design drugs that mechanistically attacked the parasites. By seeking to understand the parasite–host relationship, Cerami believed that he would be able to more rapidly determine a scientific road-map to guide his attempts to find effective chemotherapeutic agents as opposed to the empirical methodology that revealed mechanisms only secondarily. For inspiration, Cerami turned to Paul Ehrlich, whose brilliance in antiprotozoal chemotherapy he found spellbinding when, as a child, he had read the book *Microbe Hunters*. At the beginning of the twentieth century, Ehrlich discovered the first antitrypanosomal drug for the treatment of cattle in Africa, and because the disease continued to be devastating to livestock genetically evolved from European breeds, Cerami decided that one potentially exciting way to expand on Meshnick's work would be to explore trypanosome infections in cattle (a disease known as Nagana).[24]

Underpinning much of Cerami's scientific work in the 1970s, and which gave rise to his trailblazing status in translational medicine, was an emphasis on free radical oxidation reactions.[25] In particular, he advanced the theory that oxidative stress caused damage to cells and DNA and was a major factor responsible in aging. Intriguingly, it was also thought at the time that oxidative stress was involved in the mode of action of a number of existing microbial drugs. Cerami is fond of saying that "there is no magic sauce" to the discipline of translational medicine: that it is a complex, painstakingly difficult process, which requires a continuous intellectual investment to master the large number of disciplines necessary to understand the diverse themes of the physiology of aging, the defects in molecular and cellular processes, knowledge of how the body fights infection, and the genetics of hemoglobinopathies.[26] Cerami believed strongly that it was the responsibility of the scientist to work for the benefit of society, and eschewing a singular specialism for fear of becoming intellectually quarantined, he used translational medicine as a vehicle for continuing his scientific education.[27] But there was no grand plan: the objective was to use basic science and the tools that were available at the time to understand the disease process. He did not see himself as being intellectually superior or some type of highfalutin mastermind, but he did have common sense and an inquiring mind, qualities that the immunologist Peter Medawar believed were essential to being a good scientist.[28] Science is a knowledge creation endeavor, but far from being embarrassed by his lack of understanding of the complexities of cellular immunology, if Cerami did not feel entirely competent in a certain area of immunoparasitology, he used his powerful position to assemble an academic conference on the subject at RF's renowned Bellagio Study Center, on Lake Como, Italy.[29] In fact, throughout the 1980s, Cerami played an active role in advancing the discipline of parasitology in the United States and beyond. In 1983, together with the National Institutes of Health (NIH) parasitologist, Alan Sher, Cerami organized the Second Gordon Conference on "Immunological and Molecular Aspects of Parasitism," which attracted over 150 participants from across the world. He was also instrumental in establishing the world-renowned Biology of Parasitism course held every summer in the Marine Biological Laboratory in Woods Hole, Massachusetts.[30] Likewise, in his role as a teacher, he organized courses at The Rockefeller University, enquiring into medical problems that he was interested in solving, and invited experts in the field to discuss their ideas about the ways to facilitate science to help drive innovation. He was constantly trying to think of ways to harness the scientific power of The Rockefeller University's brilliant workforce to benefit society. Importantly, Cerami had a deep personal commitment to science and a well-developed taste for its adventure, excitement, and romance.[31] Similarly, he reveled in the opportunity that translational research offered to interact with other equally dedicated colleagues, including Barry Bloom, Bridget Ogilvie, and John David. He was conscious that he was not yet a fully formed theorist and researcher and that to be truly effective in science, he needed to be relevant and to develop a set of exacting attributes. In the late 1970s, he was still learning, still a student at heart.

Inspiring the members of his lab with intriguing questions relating to human biology was the pinnacle of science for Cerami, and for him, the broader the perspective, the better. To enable this scientific ideal to flourish, Cerami gathered an ecumenical group of research scientists into his lab. This collective endeavor brings to mind Lewis Thomas's depiction of the life scientific, seen at times as a lonely activity and yet communal and interdependent. If the objective is to find a single piece of truth about nature, the "whole scientific enterprise must be arranged so that the separate imaginations of different human minds must be pooled, and this is more a kind of game than a systematic business. It is in the abrupt, unaccountable aggregation of random notions, intuitions, known in science as good ideas, that the high points are made."[32] Their truly interdisciplinary composition, amalgamating in the same research environment, synthetic and organic chemists working alongside biologists, pathologists, and immunologists, helped Cerami's lab to cultivate a palpable sense of confidence that it would be possible to intervene in a disease process with a small molecule therapy—a drug.

Meshnick's first extrapolative discovery was that trypanosomes do not make heme,[33] indicating that they lacked catalase, a very important protective enzyme defense against oxidative damage. This was the "Achilles' heel" the researchers had been looking for, a structural difference between the parasite and the host enzymes that could be exploited for the development of agents to combat parasitic diseases.[34] With Cerami's background in hemoglobin metabolism, it was decided to treat the trypanosomes with a family of porphyrin complexes of free radical initiators, heme, and hematoporphyrin D, which caused the hydrogen peroxide within the parasites to fragment, killing the parasites by causing lesion-like pores in their membranes. It therefore appeared to the researchers that the organisms did not have an enzymatic means of disposing of this fatal toxic compound. The trypanocidal action of the mechanism worked so convincingly in vitro, and in mice and rats in the laboratory setting, that when the opportunity arose to study and treat cattle infected with trypanosomes at the International Laboratory for Research in Animal Diseases (ILRAD) in Nairobi, Kenya, Cerami's expectations for his first foray into the "bush" were justifiably high.

Throughout his career, Cerami had learned to trust in his insights; he cherished the sensation that came from seeing something for the first time and felt a deep emotional satisfaction when his work as a basic scientist had the capacity to link a problem to its solution. Surely now, after all the "hard, lonely work"[35] associated with science, Cerami's adhesion to rational drug design would be vindicated? Alas, when Meshnick and Cerami injected the compound into the *T. brucei*–infected cows, it set off a free radical storm causing violent convulsions and the death of the emaciated animals within fifteen minutes![36] Upon seeing the devastation caused by the compound, Cerami felt inadequate, self-diminished, and embarrassed. If that was not enough, humiliation soon followed, as very quickly a joke began to circulate among ILRAD staff. "Have you heard that those guys from New York City have developed a great diagnostic to identify trypanosome infected animals? The problem was the readout was their death."[37] The criticism and sense of failure was felt deeply by Cerami, and over the following weeks, he analyzed again and again the events that he had witnessed, asking himself what could be a possible explanation. One of the main problems with trypanosome infections is that the animals lose a considerable amount of muscle and fat—literally wasting away until their death.[38] As a child, Cerami had been introduced to the wasting condition, cachexia, through the diseases of animals on the family farm—coccidiosis in chickens and tuberculosis and brucellosis in cows. Later, his father died of cancer of the bowel, tragically undergoing severe wasting before succumbing to the malignancy. All of these images and experiences were spiraling around in his mind when one morning, while examining some cattle in the ILRAD corral, Cerami developed a bout of severe gastritis and decided to sit down among the trypanosome-infected cattle and wait for the stomachache to subside.

Part of the intimacy of being in nature, far away from the built environment, is that a heightening of the senses can occur that allows the natural world to come more clearly into focus. Cerami had been brought up in rural isolation, where awareness was turned outward, concentrated on the immediate countryside. A part of him would always be in bucolic New Jersey; the landscapes, influences, and images he grew up among were the ones he continued to return to in his mind. Living on the land carried with it an attendant necessity to be more conscious of what was going on in nature—after all, on the farm, he was the custodian of the animals, and they in turn sustained his family's well-being. Now, looking around the corral at the cattle, and as the pain in his belly began to recede, Cerami's mind focused once more on the acerbic joke that his compound would be useful for identifying infected animals. This was, upon reflection, an interesting idea, especially as when he had given the drug to noninfected cattle, they had shown no ill effects whatsoever. Just as intriguingly, the infected cows, far from being inundated, had very few parasites in their body—this anomaly posed an intriguing biological conundrum for Cerami: how could so few parasites cause such a catastrophic weight loss and death in a comparatively large animal? The answer gave Cerami his eureka moment in translational medicine. "It hit me like a brick. It was because the cow was killing itself, and that it was an inappropriate reaction to a few parasites. This meant that the parasite was not the problem. The problem is that the body is making something that is causing the cachexia."[39] This proposed immunogenic response led Cerami, while still sitting in the dusty corral, to construct a theory that would profoundly influence the science of immunology and the future of drug discovery.

As a child, Cerami had been told that the wasting disease cachexia that affected his family's farm animals was a result of the tumors or organisms using the body of the host for their own growth. At The Rockefeller University, Cerami began to question this explanation after having observed anemia and cachexia in different species due to diverse organisms and tumors of disparate etiology. "I hypothesized," reasoned Cerami, "that during the course of evolution, animals adopted primitive defense systems, which could none-specifically kill invaders. Sometimes, in the case of the cow, the response was out of proportion to the threat. The wild animals of Africa had further evolved and adjusted their response to the challenge appropriate to the invasion of the trypanosomes."[40] Cerami's flash of insight was given added biological coherence by the findings of ILRAD veterinarians who had studied wild African antelopes with similar levels of parasitemia as his cattle but did not go on to develop the wasting disease cachexia. This observation had the effect of confirming his cause-and-effect rationale and acted as an intellectual springboard to his intuitive ability to observe the pattern of disease taking place around him and then leap ahead of the scientific rationale on a self-confessed "guess."[41] Thus, the scientific expedition to Kenya, which had begun with a catastrophic failure illustrating the shortcomings of Cerami's theory of rational drug design,[42] had now been transformed into a search for a mediator responsible for cachexia. Not only that, but it held out the tantalizing possibility that if the mediator could be identified, might it be possible to prevent its action?[43] If Cerami could answer these two biological challenges, he recognized that he would have insights into the pathogenesis of many human diseases.

The German poet Hermann Hesse has written that a magic dwells in each beginning,[44] and the ten-year research program that Cerami sketched out in his mind while sitting on the parched earth of the ILRAD enclosure had emerged from the debris of a scientific failure that had left him subdued and downcast. Salvation came through a combination of courage, lateral thinking, and the ability to visualize the molecular basis of life, via which one could formulate a hypothesis to be tested by experiment. This scientific attitude exemplified the Warren ideal of the bench-to-bush and bush-to-bench dynamic.[45] In a wider context, what Cerami's early work in parasitology showed is that in the basic sciences, flashes of insight and discoveries cannot be planned. Perhaps that is why Francis Crick chose as the title of his autobiography *What Mad Pursuit*.[46] Cerami realized that the underlying biology of many diseases is not understood. From this observation, he learned the value of making bold simplifying assumptions based on the chemical validation of concepts while at the same time being critical, but not overly so, about the fit between the theory and existing pathophysiological thinking. That first visit to Kenya had, however, been instructive, demonstrating as it did the countervailing forces that operate at the boundary between basic science and the translational pathway. It also highlighted the reality that the passage of a scientific discovery can be a long and circuitous one. A laboratory, or indeed an individual, can frequently set out to pursue one concept, which can then lead to another field of inquiry, sometimes related and sometimes not. Often this is how science works—but what is key is the ability to recognize the research area of greatest potential and to stick to it. Whether it was the result of luck, knowledge of the chemical biology of life, or intuition, one of Cerami's recognized talents as a biomedical scientist was amazing prescience: he had the vision to see what the next experiment should be to move a hypothesis forward, and just as importantly, he had at his disposal a talented collection of early career physician-scientists eager to carry out his scientific program.[47]

By the time Cerami arrived back in New York City, he had designed a research project for his graduate student, Carol Rouser, that he hoped would be able to find the clue needed to unravel the biochemistry of cachexia. Unconsciously, he was moving into a field that did not yet exist. Carol Rouser's background was in synthetic organic chemistry, and she had joined the lab in 1976, cutting her experimentalist teeth investigating how glucose affects lens crystallins in the eye. For Rouser, this new project was an altogether different undertaking that reflected Cerami's experiences in Kenya and his wider thinking on the etiology of the diseases. His finding that trypanosomes do not have catalase and so were very sensitive to oxidative damage with perforins and other free radicals excited him in its own right. Tellingly, he also thought that chemically, this peroxide element might be extended to other diseases that were not parasitic, and he arrived at this belief because of one of the effects of trypanosomiasis is anemia. "Many chronic diseases," Rouser recognized, "like cancer or rheumatoid arthritis are associated with anemia. Tony thought that possibly a similar kind of mechanism, free radical–based damage, was causing anemia in both cases. Of course, leading on from this chronic anemia is cachexia, with the accompanying loss of appetite, loss of weight, and generally feeling awful."[48] Rather than using mice and rats as Steve Meshnick had done, Carol Rouser found that a better model for studying anemia and trypanosomiasis was in rabbits. In an attempt to reproduce the same conditions encountered by Cerami and Meshnick in Nairobi, the rabbits had a very low parasitemia and, after infection, quickly developed severe wasting. Rouser began by analyzing the anemia associated with the cachexia of this condition. This revealed that the main reasons for the anemia were an increased rate of red blood cell removal[49] and a decreased rate of production of new red blood cells in the infected animals, which led her to make this far-reaching observation. "The thing that struck me more than anything else was that when I would take the blood from these rabbits and centrifuged it to separate the red blood cells from the white blood cells and parasites, the serum that was above the red blood cells was very cloudy and the sicker the animals became, the cloudier the serum was."[50] That the straw-colored plasma above the red blood cells and buffy coat was opaque suggested to Rouser that it was due to lipid droplets, indicating that "there was too much fat in the serum, and the animals became extremely lipemic. I became quite fascinated with this phenomenon of the extra lipids and the discovery that the animals were not clearing triglycerides from their blood very well."[51] During the course of Rouser's investigations, she was able to demonstrate that the plasma of the infected rabbits was extremely lipemic due to the visible accumulation of very low-density lipoprotein in the plasma. Further studies revealed that the lipemia was the result of the loss of the enzyme lipoprotein lipase, which is responsible for the breakdown of triglycerides in the blood, allowing free fatty acids to be taken up by endothelial cells and transported out of the bloodstream to muscle and cells, where they could be metabolized. This penetrating observation was the key to beginning to unravel the molecular basis of cachexia.

Laboring round-the-clock in the light-deprived, subterranean lab throughout the winter months, Carol Rouser discussed her experiments with another member of Cerami's team, Eileen Mahoney, who had a background in lipid biochemistry gained while studying in the laboratory of cell biologist Zanvil Cohn.[52] At around this time, the talented Rouser decided to leave Cerami's lab to continue her doctoral thesis with William A. Scott, a lipid biochemist in Cohn's laboratory. Carol Rouser's decision to leave his laboratory was difficult for Cerami to accept as he knew her to be productive, tenacious, and insightful. "One day Carol said to me, 'you don't really know anything about lipid metabolism' and I confessed, that I didn't know a lot about anything, but that I was willing to read, to learn. But it wasn't enough; she decided that it was too difficult a project for a PhD thesis and chose to pursue her studies in another lab."[53]

From the start of his career, Cerami became aware of an inescapable dilemma of pursuing a life in science: that creative resources are often overstretched and that, intellectually, researchers are in the dark much of the time. Nevertheless, progress was made by thinking in terms of concepts, trying to deduce biological associations, occupying the viewpoint of the wide-angled lens, and talking to experts in different but related fields. It was to Cerami's good fortune that ideas could be resuscitated or usefully deconstructed by the insights of colleagues who had succeeded in building The Rockefeller University's enviable reputation for scientific cooperation and collegiality (the mistrustful Gerald Edelman excepted). Scientifically, often the best conversations and most enlightening insights can come from speaking to colleagues in different disciplines. Consequently, if Cerami was grappling with an aspect of innate immunity, he could simply walk into Henry Kunkel's office, editor of the journal *Experimental Medicine*, and talk to him (admittedly Kunkel was notoriously laconic), or if he wanted to refine his thinking on the heme units of malaria pigment, he could speak to William Trager, the scientist who first cultured the malaria parasite. The laboratories of The Rockefeller University abounded with specialists, and one of Cerami's colleagues, Nobel Prize winner Bruce Merrifield, an expert on peptide synthesis, was always on hand to offer advice over a problem-solving lunch on how to make new molecules. In fact, as well as being a beneficiary of this problem-solving nexus, Cerami was a contributor to the ideal, and being able to put people together to elucidate biomedical problems was seen by some as his major talent as a laboratory leader.[54] It was also widely acknowledged that Cerami was good with young scholars in his lab, and the tropical health physician Keith McAdam, another founder member of the GND family, understood the creative dynamics being played out at the work bench. "Tony made young researchers feel that their science was important, he allowed them to 'own' their work—he gave them the limelight."[55] Mostly his management style worked, but occasionally, as with the dedicated if disillusioned Rouser, it did not. Having come from a small private liberal arts school, Rouser, a self-confessed "science nerd," lacked experience in high-level research or a specialism and, as a consequence, perhaps needed more mentoring, guidance, and pedagogic support than The Rockefeller University customarily gave their graduate students.[56]

Philosophically, Cerami found that learning from failures[57] was the most productive way to live with scientific unknowns because it was through this method that critical thinking developed, allowing him to make new insights and discoveries. As a scientific theorist, Cerami saw the world from a chemist's point of view. This was both his strength and also a source of potential weakness. On the one hand, it galvanized him and put him ahead of the game with regard to providing a chemical validation of concept, but it could also be an impediment to his envisioning life from the perspective of cellular physiology—where the thinking was more in terms of *networks*. Carol Rouser was not alone in recognizing Cerami's pioneering status in identifying the deleterious effects of free radicals,[58] but free radical oxidation reactions did not explain the specific phenomenon Rouser set out to explore—anemia in chronic disease—or her discovery of hyperlipidemia.[59] What was certain, however, was that Rouser's observation that the rabbits were lipemic due to the loss of the enzyme lipoprotein lipase was the signal finding that persuaded Cerami to change track and hypothesize that it was a hormone or proinflammatory signaling protein that was released due to the infection that perturbed normal metabolic functions and caused the well-known weight loss and wasting associated with cancer and trypanosomiasis.[60] It was clear that study of the loss of this enzyme in response to invasion would be a good biomarker to identify and isolate the mediator.[61] It was at this time that Cerami turned the search for this mediator over to Masanobu "Nobu" Kawakami, a dedicated and talented postdoctoral fellow in his laboratory.

Nobu Kawakami was put in charge of the project because he knew about lipoproteins, having contributed to the development of an assay of glucocorticoids in human blood in his native Tokyo and then later in the laboratory of Dr. DeWitt Goodman in Columbia University, New York, where he worked on a vitamin D carrier protein.[62] Also, Cerami liked to employ medics because they came with an understanding of biological mechanisms, and he could utilize their gargantuan work ethic, but in Nobu Kawakami, he had found a researcher capable of extraordinary feats of dedication and labor. He was accurate, he was capable, and Cerami came to think of Kawakami as both a friend and a "human machine." Having extensively reviewed the literature of metabolic derangements in a variety of exogenous and endogenous geneses, including cancer, infections, and allergic diseases, Kawakami and Cerami quickly ruled out the continuing use of rabbits infected with trypanosomes and instead chose a mouse model of endotoxemia. Endotoxin or lipopolysaccharide (LPS) causes catastrophic metabolic disturbances and death when injected into humans and other animals.[63] The decision to change the animal model was based on a research paper that Kawakami discovered during one of his nocturnal pilgrimages in The Rockefeller University library.[64] The paper noted that there were two strains of mice that were closely related. One *responder* mouse, C3H/HeN, was sensitive to endotoxin (causing the death of the animal), and the other *nonresponder*, C3H/HeJ, was resistant and not killed by the administration of LPS.

The researchers performed a simple experiment showing that the administration of endotoxin to the sensitive mouse (N) led to a decrease in lipoprotein lipase, whereas the administration of endotoxin to the resistant mouse (J) did not.[65] Their hypothesis was that if they took sera from the sensitive mouse that had been injected with endotoxin and gave them to the resistant mouse, there would be a suppression of lipoprotein lipase—signaling the presence of their destructive mediator. Kawakami, a poet laureate of laboratory experiments, describes the excitement felt in one of those moments when hypothesis-driven science successfully reveals one of nature's secrets. "I was thrilled in one midnight session when the scintillation counter started to print out very low counts, which meant that a new mediator was being made by the [N mouse] that could suppress lipoprotein lipase in the J mouse. . . . With this experiment we could prove that endotoxin induced the production of a mediator that could suppress lipoprotein lipase."[66] To fulfill his childhood dream of wanting to help sick people, Cerami knew that the next decisive issue that needed to be addressed was the source of the endogenous mediator.

Nobu brought an intensity and passion to the search and was guided by what he described as Cerami's "excellent insights into the molecular interactions, which bring biological and clinical meaning."[67] Observations drive progress and, as macrophages are key immune cells, Cerami suggested to Kawakami that macrophages might be a good place to start the search as Zanvil Cohn's lab had been studying the scavenger cells for over a decade.[68] Cohn and Cerami were friends, and Cohn, the founder of modern macrophage biology, carried out innovative investigations that revealed the role of these large scavenger cells that engulf and consume invaders, including bacteria. Macrophages are central to innate immunity and to inflammation, and beginning in 1963, Cohn was to spend the next thirty years using this crucial cell as a tool for important discoveries in cell biology.[69] The modern-day concept of the laboratory without walls originated at The Rockefeller University, where there were no departments, and the scientific connective thread of cooperation came via informal conversations and collaborations. Cohn collaborated for many years with the biologist Jim Hirsh (who introduced Cerami to Warren), whose long-term interest was in white blood cells called phagocytes that kill invading microbes. So, Nobu Kawakami was indeed in good hands, and he made the most of his relationship with Cohn's lab to understand the cell biology of macrophages. Very soon, Cerami and Kawakami were able to show that the incubation of peritoneal macrophages from sensitive mice with endotoxin produced a mediator that could suppress lipoprotein lipase in resistant mice. This observation was a big step forward, and the researchers were now able to produce the mediator in vitro and induce the mediator by adding endotoxin.[70]

In his quest to find a simpler bioassay for the mediator, Cerami dispatched Kawakami to Baltimore to work with Phil Pekala in Dan Lane's laboratory at Johns Hopkins Medical School. Over the following months, the devoted Kawakami found little time for Reiko, his wife, and two children as he was working on macrophages at the weekend in New York and on adipocytes, a specialized cell for the storage of fat, during the week in Baltimore. But his dedication paid off. Using a special fibroblast cell line, 3T3-L1, that had been induced to form fat cells, the addition of the mediator led to a specific turning off of Lipoprotein lipase LPL (a water-soluble enzyme) and other enzymes responsible for fatty acid synthesis and uptake.[71] The development of the 3T3-L1 cell assay was an excellent bioassay for their defining breakthrough—the isolation of the mediator. In addition, the researchers were able to demonstrate that the bioactive material that they introduced in macrophages inhibited red blood cell production in vitro.[72] This observation was particularly pleasing to Kawakami, "since it was the phenomenon of decreased red cell production in rabbits infected with trypanosomes that gave the initial clue of hyperlipidaemia that allowed us to go forward."[73]

For Cerami, almost nothing was more exciting than the thrill of discovery, especially after a long and confusing search. The sense of failure that he had felt while prostrate in the corral in Kenya was now replaced with one of immense satisfaction by the discovery that a single protein, whose primary function was the regulation of immune cells, was causing all the problems associated with cachexia. Of course, other researchers had thought of the possibility of a mediator long before Cerami entered the field, but the necessary technology, obsessive drive, and the conceptual insights were not in place until he came along. Medical research begins with efforts to understand how living systems actually work and from there moves on to figure out when they are broken.[74] Understanding the mechanism of cachexia had proved a tremendous challenge, but once the researchers had the ability to induce a mediator with many activities that had been associated with anemia and cachexia, Cerami, with customary taxonomic flair, decided to name the protein *cachectin*.

The new decade of the 1980s witnessed Cerami's attempt to unravel one of the most profound processes in immunology. In considering the role of natural selection—leading to unlikely and intricate mechanisms—on our genetic makeup, Cerami believed that cachectin's primary function was the regulation of immune cells and that its role evolved as a mechanism to combat the invasion of an infection caused by a virus or bacteria. He saw it as a beautiful and efficient way of killing something that is foreign in the body but that it proved too efficient and, in certain circumstances, even lethal. "The body responds to any injury or inflammation as if it were an infection. The effect is so powerful it produces ripples throughout the body, killing everything around the infection, including perfectly healthy tissue far beyond the area of the original wound or trauma."[75] Self–nonself discrimination is the main function of the immune system, but what Cerami found did not fit into the conceptual matrix of accepted immunological thinking. For him, cachectin was a highly proinflammatory protein responsible for destroying everything in the area where a trauma is occurring but that it has a problem of overkill. Via the application of basic knowledge, Cerami unraveled a profound process in immunology and discovered one of the great paradoxes in nature. Cachectin is the solution *and* the problem.[76]

Every effort was now concentrated on proving that the existence of the mediator could cause metabolic change.[77] Within a short time, Kawakami and Cerami were able to identify a protein with an apparent molecular weight of 70 kDa (a kilodalton is a unit of molecular mass consisting of 1,000 daltons) that was made by macrophages in response to endotoxin, malaria pigment, trypanosomes, and a number of other agents that signaled a pathological invasion of the mammalian body.[78] Being able to mimic an effect by giving this mediator *without* the presence an infection gave Cerami "a sense of triumph, as we had been able to describe the genius of evolution: a single protein with all that power."[79] Alas, to Cerami's growing frustration, the clinical significance of the mediator was not readily accepted by leading specialists across medical disciplines. "They thought," Kawakami remembers, "this factor may have some role only in infections or endotoxemia but not in the wide variety of situations, even though we showed many agents including immune complex stimulate macrophages to produce this factor."[80] Undeterred, in 1981, Cerami and Kawakami wrote a legally compelling patent describing their work on the characteristics of *cachectin* and the roles that it played in many pathological conditions.[81] The researchers also proposed that the neutralization of the human self-antigen *cachectin* by monoclonal antibodies would be beneficial in a number of human diseases and inflammatory conditions, including shock, cachexia, and rheumatoid arthritis.

Energized by the discovery of the danger of the deregulated production of *cachectin*, Cerami was now determined to find out exactly what the mediator was, clone it, and, using new technology, make monoclonal antibodies to reverse the metabolic upheaval that characterizes chronic inflammation. Just then, with mystifying exactitude, disaster struck. Masanobu Kawakami, his faithful, brilliant, and unbending scientific collaborator, announced that he was leaving The Rockefeller University to return to Japan. Unsurprisingly, Kawakami's long-suffering wife, Reiko, and two sons wanted to spend more time with Nobu, and this could only be achieved by a return to a more conventional career structure in their native Japan. Cerami made a heartfelt appeal to his friend to stay and continue on their great voyage of discovery, but Nobu was resolute. Why oh why could Cerami not retain his most valued researchers? For a passing moment, Cerami thought that his research project might come to symbolize the life cycle of the Japanese cherry blossom and fall at its moment of perfection. Possibly it was true that the journey from initial failure, rather like a persistent trope in the novels of the Japanese writer Haruki Murakami, is through darkness before arriving at the light. In the early 1980s, Cerami now stood as a lone scientific voice suggesting that the protein that he had discovered played a role in the detrimental effects of acute and chronic inflammation.[82] Fortunately, overcoming adversity was very much in his DNA.

8 · CACHECTIN—TUMOR NECROSIS FACTOR

Essentially as a scientist, as a group leader, you are the captain of a pirate ship. You have got this motley crew; some of them will jump ship, some will try to steal your stuff, some will try to cut your throat, but on balance if you can take that ship out and get the gold off the Spaniards, they'll stick around you.
—Greg Winter, Nobel Laureate in Chemistry, 2018

Infection is an important driver of evolution. Tony Cerami witnessed this biological reality early in life as his childhood coincided with the introduction of antibiotics and chemotherapeutic agents into livestock production and animal feeds. This allowed him to observe that the epidemic catastrophes, which only months previously had decimated entire populations of farm animals, could be largely controlled and even eradicated. The powerful impression formed by these observations determined the direction of his life scientific, much of which concentrated on the evolution of the human biological system to damage itself and his biomedical efforts to stop or limit this self-destruction.[1]

Humans have existed on earth for some 200,000 years,[1] and millennia before the invention of antibiotics, the body evolved a mechanism of dealing with invaders, whether viral, bacterial, or parasitical. Understanding this complex response to infection was the driving force that led Cerami to the discovery of cachectin, a molecule responsible for several destructive aspects of chronic inflammation.[2] In a letter to Joshua Lederberg, president of The Rockefeller University, Cerami described the biological rationale that underpinned his research. "Evidently, cachectin is part of an early warning system of the immune system to mobilize energy for combating invasion. This advantageous system becomes deleterious, however, if the immune system does not remove the invader. In this situation, the animal continues to mobilize energy until all stores are depleted."[3] The discovery that endogenous proteins caused disease marked a profound moment in immunology and formed the conceptual foundation upon which Cerami's contribution to translational medicine was built.

One morning in 1982, Cerami took a phone call from his good friend Ernest Beutler. "Ernie" Beutler was a renowned hematologist who specialized in red blood cell metabolism and the causes of anemia at the Scripps Research Institute in La Jolla, California. Ernie wanted to know if it would be possible for Tony to find a position for his son, Bruce, who was a medical resident (Department of Neurology) at the University of Texas Southwestern Medical Center in Dallas and would in the near future need to gain research experience at the laboratory bench. Ever eager to please a generous and trusted friend, and one who also had a reputation helping young people develop their scientific careers, Cerami's reply was, "Sure, ask him to get in contact." Not content with merely helping his son, Cerami's admiration for Ernie was such that he seriously explored the possibility of also finding a permanent position for him in New York City.[4]

During the long humid summer days of 1982, work in the lab on cachectin accelerated and began to crystallize. Nguyen Le Trang was making good progress on the isolation of the protein but, as Cerami indicated in a letter to his friend and former colleague, "Nobu" Kawakami, a vital element had been lost when he returned to Japan: "I would give anything right now to be able to have a new Nobu Kawakami in our midst."[5] That same week, a letter of introduction arrived on Cerami's desk from Bruce Beutler in Dallas, Texas. "I have recently spoken with my father, who informed me of the availability of a post-doctoral training fellowship in your laboratory. Both prior to and during the years of my clinical training, I acquired fairly broad laboratory experience ... my interests are quite flexible, and I believe that further exposure to biochemical techniques and reasoning would be very helpful to me. .... From what I have read of your work, and from appraisals given me by my father and others, I believe that a fellowship in your laboratory would be a very rewarding experience."[6] The following July, Beutler joined the laboratory as a research associate on a salary of $25,000 and immediately threw himself into the task at hand. In the 1970s, when the research work began, Cerami had offered Carol Rouser the academic limelight, insisting on her name appearing as first author on their breakthrough publication, but whereas Rouser had been reluctant to become the focus of attention, Beutler enthusiastically embraced the opportunity. From the outset, the personal chemistry between the two men was good. Cerami sought to nurture Bruce Beutler's talent, and their relationship was defined by acts of kindness and warmth. On March 2, 1983, while still living in Dallas, Texas, Beutler wrote a heartwarming letter to his new boss, in which, in addition to addressing the essential subjects of work and accommodation, he also enclosed an enchanting photograph of "the newest member of our family, shown at ten days of age. He is now three weeks old, and his name is Daniel Edward. I look forward to introducing you to him soon."

Two years previously, Kawakami and Cerami had defined their patent that would have important ramifications in the decades to come,[7] but they had not been able to completely purify their mediator or obtain its genetic sequence. Fred Sanger, who twice won the Nobel Prize in Chemistry, established that the character of a protein was determined by the sequence of its amino acids; Beutler, through the application of what Cerami described as "exceptional motivation"[8] and persistence, was able to isolate the protein and purify to homogeneity using the techniques of molecular biology.[9]

In the mid-1980s, microsequencing was in its infancy, but from a new isolation procedure that Beutler had devised, Cerami hoped that it would be possible to reveal the amino acid and genetic sequence of their mouse cachectin. For assistance, Cerami turned to Peter Lomedico, who ran drug discovery and development projects at the pharmaceutical company Hoffman-La Roche. Lomedico suggested that his colleague Yu-Ching Pan, who had the recently taken delivery of state-of-the-art technology, would be an ideal person to help identify the amino-terminal sequence of mouse cachectin. On his first attempt, Pan successfully sequenced the mouse cachectin. However, the initial jubilation was short-lived. When Pan searched the protein sequence databases, he observed homology between Cerami's mouse cachectin to human tumor necrosis factor (TNF) that had recently been sequenced.[10] In her insightful and eminently readable book on the proteins of cellular communication, Giamila Fantuzzi explained the evolution of the cloning of TNF thus: "Indeed, in 1984, another team happened on the same body message by taking a completely different route, yet one that still began with microbes."[11] Beguilingly, two completely separate groups had been studying different properties of the same molecule. Of course, it must be remembered that parallel discoveries are nothing new in science. Notably, in the middle of the past century when the epidemic of lung cancer was first being investigated by researchers in the United States, the United Kingdom, and beyond, all were working independently and unaware of each other's existence.[12] In fact, five papers were published in 1950 on the dangers of smoking tobacco: a codiscovery that provided the basis for what remains the single most reliably established and practical means of reducing the proportion of deaths from cancer.

Although what was *new* in this instance and a "complete surprise" to Cerami was that TNF had been discovered by Lloyd Old and his team at Memorial Sloan-Kettering Cancer Center, directly across the street from The Rockefeller University.[13] This was revelatory simply because some years earlier, Cerami was concerned that cachectin was the same as other macrophage mediator proteins that had been reported, including interleukin 1 (IL-1) and TNF. As a precaution, he had sent Nobu Kawakami to exchange their mouse cachectin for human tumor necrosis factor with Elizabeth Carswell, a close colleague of Lloyd Old's at the Sloan-Kettering Institute. In the Rockefeller's 3T3-L1 assay, the Sloan-Kettering TNF had no cachectin activity; likewise, the Rockefeller's cachectin exhibited no activity in the Sloan-Kettering TNF bioassay. Why these experiments did not work is unclear, but it led Nobo Kawakami to reflect wearily, "It certainly would have saved a lot of time and effort."[14] When Old and Cerami subsequently discussed this anomaly the consensus arrived at was that negative experiments did not count for much.[15] Lloyd Old, a California-born physician, whose motto was *in vivo veritas* (in the living thing there is proof), was widely recognized as a leading figure in modern tumor immunology,[16] and he shared Cerami's unwavering dedication to translating basic research in animals into clinical research in human diseases. Old had been studying proteins released by macrophages in their biological resistance against tumors, and named the protein tumor necrosis factor (TNF). The history of tumor necrosis activity dated back to the end of the nineteenth century when William B. Coley, a surgeon at Memorial Hospital, New York City, injected a streptococcal potion into a patient with inoperable cancer. This method resulted in the disappearance of some patients' tumors.[17] Attempts to utilize this approach had variable results because of the inherent toxicity (lethal shock) from injecting cancer patients with bacteria. Almost a century later, Lloyd Old and his group injected mice and rabbits with Coley-type bacteria, which produced a substance endowed with the ability to destroy cancer.[18] They reasoned that lipopolysaccharide was inducing macrophages to produce a protein that could kill tumor cells and that that activity could be separated from lethal shock activity. Their results with purified TNF and later recombinant human TNF were quite dramatic in some mouse tumor models. The problem was that beyond the tumor shrinkage, there was also extensive damage to other organs.

The biological revelation that cachectin and TNF were the same multipotent protein led Bruce Beutler to experience a period of introspection and deep reflection at the sheer unknowability of the finding. In another remarkable historical coincidence, protein chemist Barbara Sherry was visiting Cerami's lab on the very day Beutler discovered that cachectin and tumor necrosis factor were one and the same molecule. Barbara Sherry began her professional life as a basic scientist and, under Cerami's mentorship, succeeded in bridging the divide to become a translational scientist, first at The Rockefeller University and later at other biomedical institutions. In fact, Sherry was in New York to attend an interview with Cerami for a postgraduate position, and during the course of the day, she was introduced to Beutler. It was a memorable occasion: "We were in a small room," recalled Sherry, "but we were not talking and Bruce's head was bowed." Unexpectedly, Beutler shifted his gaze, and looking across at Barbara Sherry declared, "I'm really sorry, but I've just found out something that could easily be the best thing in my life, or it can destroy my life."[19]

Statistically, it was an extreme chance event and an extraordinary scientific coincidence that two labs situated directly across the street from each other were studying different properties of the same molecule. The juxtaposition was clear and understandable: had the work of the Laboratory of Medical Biochemistry been preempted, or was a whole new area of immunology about to be opened up for investigation that the Sloan-Kettering group had not considered? Cerami had been a lone voice in thinking that cachectin was a cytokine that led to metabolic derangements such as anemia and inflammation, and throughout the following months, Cerami, with Beutler, published a series of articles that changed the whole thinking surrounding TNF as an anticancer agent.

In a review article entitled "Cachectin and Tumor Necrosis Factor as Two Sides of the Same Coin,"[20] Cerami and Beutler examined the antitumor and the inflammatory effect of "cachectin/TNF." They reported that there were many clinical benefits in blocking cachectin in patients who were at risk of shock, inflammation, and the effects of infection. Previously, researchers had not been thinking about the molecule in terms of host inflammatory response. They also reported the initial isolation of TNF, and its use as an anticancer agent "was predicted on the assumption that a means of retaining the tumor necrotic effect of endotoxin, while dispensing with its toxic properties, had been found. It now appears, however, that cachectin (TNF) is the principal mediator of both exotoxin-induced shock and tumor necrosis."[21] Conterminously, the researchers presented a paper entitled, "Cachectin: The Dark Side of Tumor Necrosis Factor," at a symposium at Cold Spring Harbor,[22] which struck a resonant chord both with the scientific community and with the wider public. Under the headline "Anticancer Substance Reveals Its Dark Side," a New York Times article[23] juxtaposed the countervailing scientific interpretations in terms of bright and dark sides of the human body's reaction to disease, with the bright side being TNF as a possible weapon against cancer and the dark side being cachectin—a powerful natural substance that could have a deadly role. So a picture began to evolve of a protein with a known string of 157 amino acids that had two different names and two widely divergent interpretations of its biological role.

Science is a human construct, and the precise chemical characteristics of cachectin/ TNF were determined during an intriguing period of medical discourse in the United States. The modern war against cancer began in the United States in 1970 with the publication of the Yarborough report, which advanced a set of recommendations and a strategy for the "means and measures necessary to facilitate success in the treatment, cure and elimination of cancer—at the earliest possible date."[24] President Richard Nixon signed the National Cancer Act into law on December 23, 1971, with a propitious wish: "I hope in the years ahead we will look back on this action today as the most significant action taken during my administration."[25] 1971 was also the year that Lloyd Old, Elizabeth Carswell, and colleagues discovered TNF, and over the following decade, Genentech and other biotech companies were gathering their resources to find the elusive "cure for cancer" that Senator Ralph W. Yarborough had memorably initiated. However, Cerami and Beutler's findings contradicted the cancer-killing role of the cytokine, and Cerami began to actively campaign against its therapeutic use, which led to much personal and scientific condemnation. Nonetheless, he believed that the administration of cachectin/TNF would lead to biological damage and death in patients with cancer and that, far from being an anticancer drug, he believed it "was an anti-living drug."[26] On one occasion, while giving a presentation on cachectin in Belgium, Cerami was criticized by a member of the audience of being a jealous scientist and guilty of trying to ruin the efforts of the emergent biotechnology industry to find a treatment for cancer. Yet far from seeking to diminish the therapeutic impetus of the embryonic industry, Cerami was being realistic about the future, seeing the great potential for blocking the activities of cachectin/TNF, which was responsible for so many inflammatory diseases. Cerami's vision for the forthcoming role of biotechnology was not the administration of TNF but rather immunization against its biological impacts.

Cerami and Beutler felt so strongly about the potential deleterious effects of TNF on patients with cancer that in June 1985, they wrote a cautionary letter to Samuel Ackerman, director of the Division of Biologics and Investigative New Drugs at the National Institutes of Health in Bethesda, Maryland, stating,

> It has come to our attention that clinical studies of tumor necrosis factor (TNF), administered as an antineoplastic agent, may soon be in progress in this country. In this regard, we feel obliged to inform you of the results of our own studies of this factor and its actions in vivo, some of which have not yet appeared in literature. . . . Of particular interest, we have noted that TNF is one of the principal mediators of the endotoxin-induced shock. When mice are passively immunized against tumor necrosis factor, they develop a marked resistance to the lethal effect of endotoxin. We expect that administration of large quantities of tumor necrosis factor might, of itself, precipitate a shock state. . . . While TNF may, at appropriate doses, prove to be of benefit as an antineoplastic agent, we believe that great caution must be exercised in administering it to human subject. . . . Given the large differences in endotoxin sensitivity that exist between species, it is possible that certain animals (e.g., rats and mice) are relatively resistant to the effects of the hormone, and may provide poor models for the prediction of TNF in humans.[27]

During the same month, they also wrote a letter in a similar vein to Karl Pinsky of the Biological Response Modifiers Program, Frederick Cancer Research Facility in Maryland.[28] Cerami's objective in writing these letters was to take TNF out of the field of anticancer agents and place the cytokine firmly in the field of inflammation.

One of the diseases that concentrated Cerami's mind from the very beginning of his work on cachectin was shock, the life-threatening condition that can damage multiple organs irreparably. Unravelling the causes of shock had blunted the wits of researchers for a generation. What was known was that a sudden and dramatic reduction in blood pressure can cause the condition. The most familiar form is anaphylactic shock, which can lead to an overproduction of histamine by mast cells. Low levels of histamine are important to host defense, but the supercharged release of large amounts, as happens when the victim is allergic to insect stings, causes shock and respiratory failure.[29] Infections that run out of control are the origin of another deadly form of shock, called septic shock. Unfortunately, we understand only the most basic rudiments of why most diseases occur, and for still unknown reasons, a localized infection can evolve into a generalized inflammatory response called sepsis, and when sepsis gets out of control, septic shock ensues.[30] Severe sepsis is one of the most common killers in the United States today, after cardiovascular disease and cancer, and millions of people die every year all

over the world of septic shock. As we have seen, Cerami's method of seeking to understand the causes of septic shock (including weight loss, plunging blood pressure,
and trauma) and how he came to discover cachectin was via the administration of
endotoxin to laboratory animals. Having developed a method to experimentally
induce endotoxic shock, Cerami now turned his attentions to the possibility of
being able to prevent the disease.

Work that Cerami had initiated almost a decade before was now blossoming,
presenting new and intriguing interpretations of the role of cytokines in the
immune system's armamentarium. In a lodestar 1985 paper published in *Science*,[31]
Cerami, Beutler, and Ian Milsark reported that blocking the activity of cachectin/
TNF in mice with a "highly specific polyclonal rabbit antiserum" offered significant protection. Whereas only 50 percent of the mice receiving the endotoxin
lipopolysaccharide survived, all of the animals in which the researchers had neutralized cachectin/TNF prior to injection of endotoxin lived.[32] This finding led
the scientists to state that the "data suggests that cachectin/TNF is one of the
principal mediators of the lethal effect of endotoxin."[33] In a prelude to the publication of the article, Cerami wrote a compelling accompanying letter to Dr. Ruth
Kulstad, senior editor at the journal in which he stated that the "possibility of treating patients with endotoxic shock by passive immunization with antibodies to
cachectin/TNF opens an exciting new approach to the management of shock."
The letter closed on a note of circumspection. "The potential commercial interest
in this report, obliges us to request that the paper not be sent to scientists with
principal interests in biotechnology companies."

When Kevin Tracey, a young neurosurgeon working across the street from The
Rockefeller University, at Cornell University Medical College, read the paper in
Science, he found it "tantalizing."[34] Tracey was in fact part of another Cerami initiative launched jointly by The Rockefeller University and Cornell University Medical School. In order to better understand the concerns of the medical profession
and with his focus on finding therapies for unmet human needs, Cerami was constantly looking for ways to collaborate with research-minded clinicians. His desire
to fuse laboratory research to clinical practice was matched by G. Tom Shires,
chairman of the Department of Surgery at Cornell. Shires was one of the leading
surgeons in the United States, and his research on the physiology and therapy of
shock changed the practice of medicine.[35] Shires's vision was to provide the new
generation of surgeons with time to develop and explore research skills in a laboratory setting that would provide biological insights into the diseases and infections that they would later treat in operating theaters.[36] Tracey's fascination with
Cerami and Beutler's paper was informed by a tragedy that he had recently witnessed. One of his patients, a young girl, had been scalded by boiling water, burning over 75 percent of her body. The damage to the infant was so great that her
immune system went into overdrive, but in an attempt to destroy the invading
bacteria, it also severely damaged her lungs, kidneys, and heart through a disease
pathway known as severe sepsis.[37] The child subsequently died in Tracey's arms;[38]

consumed by the need to understand the causes of shock and severe sepsis and to develop treatments for these life-threatening diseases, he sought answers through experiments at the bench. Working in Steve Lowry's laboratory, Tracey sought to understand the reasons that led to the rapid demise of his patient through the line of thinking articulated by the article in *Science*, in which the authors had recorded that blocking the activity of cachectin/TNF in mice conferred a significant protection against the lethal effects of a bacterial toxin. Therefore, reasoned Tracey, it seemed probable that TNF might be dangerous not only to the bacteria but also to the host. This led him to hypothesize that the body's supposed defender might have been responsible for his patient's septic shock and death.[39] To study this possibility, he set up a rodent intensive care unit on the sixth floor of the Cornell Medical College and immediately began collaborating with Cerami and Beutler on a career-defining research program.

Cerami's focus on benefiting patients in a tangible and therapeutic way came through his ability to nurture and mentor talent. And in Tracey and Beutler, he had recruited two outstanding early career scientists who had found their calling. Beutler would work sixteen-hour days every weekend to make 1 milligram of recombinant human cachectin/TNF, which, at the time, was the entire world supply, and on Monday mornings, Tracey would infuse the serum into a rat. "Looking back, it was an amazing time," recalls Tracey, "Bruce and I would walk across the campus and he would have the cachectin in an ice bucket. One morning I asked him, 'Why do you have a lid on the bucket?' His reply was, 'To protect the cachectin from the evil light of the sun.'"[40] Their experiments produced a "game changing"[41] publication in *Science* that became one of the most highly cited articles on TNF[42] with Tracey as first author, Beutler as second author, and Cerami as final contributor. They reported that when recombinant human cachectin (tumor necrosis factor) was infused into rats in quantities similar to those produced endogenously in response to endotoxin, it caused hypotension, metabolic acidosis, homoconcentration, and death within minutes to hours as a result of respiratory arrest. The paper marked a watershed in the medical history of the molecule, proving beyond doubt that the original belief that TNF could be used as a cancer therapeutic was a delusion, showing categorically that TNF was a highly dangerous molecule that needed to be blocked and not used as a treatment. Indeed, with the passage of time, it became clear that TNF promoted the production of a number of other cytokines and mediators. Cytokines are the mainstay of the immune system; they deliver their messages to target cells by binding to specific receptors,[43] but as Cerami et al. had conclusively shown, cachectin/TNF could both kill cells and protect them from death. The destructive force of the molecule seemed contradictory: why would the immune system make a protein that kills the patient?[44] The answer to this evolutionary conundrum lay in the *amount* of TNF produced. Clearly, low-level production of TNF is an essential part of the immune response to infection; as long as the amount of TNF is regulated and held within the nontoxic range, the patient benefits, but if it is unregulated and overproduced, it is toxic.

Another enigma accompanying the biological function of the molecule relates to its confusing and competing nomenclatures. Did the term *cachectin* and its association to cachexia more accurately reflect the disease process or was tumor necrosis factor (TNF) a better classification as it conjures up the idea of cell death? While Cerami was focused on establishing a clearer understanding of the mechanisms and pathways that mediate disease, in contrast, clinical practice has always been limited by its inability to differentiate clinical, biochemical, and pathological abnormalities that accompany a disease from those events actually responsible for mediating a disease process.[45] As the U.S. physician and writer Lewis Thomas pointed out in 1944, diagnosis of most human disease provides only "insecure and temporary conceptions."[46] Be that as it may, by the end of the 1980s, for reasons that may have been as much to do with the need for a uniform classification within the scientific literature as with morphological characteristics, the molecule increasingly became known as tumor necrosis factor alpha (TNFa) or TNF, and the taxonomy "cachectin" progressively disappeared. This was despite Cerami and his scientific collaborators having succeeded in taking TNF out of the field of anti-cancer agents and establishing it incontestably in the etiology of inflammation. There are many misnomers in medical classification (acoustic neuroma, sebaceous cyst, pyogenic granuloma and even interleukin 6 [IL-6], which was once termed *hybridoma growth factor*—yes, it does that, but it is not its most important activity). However, unfortunately for Cerami's renown in the world of discovery science, TNF remains a definitive exemplar of taxonomic inaccuracy. What is indisputable, however, is that the fundamental insight that a molecule produced by the immune system is both necessary and sufficient to cause inflammation was proved by Tony Cerami and other researchers in the Laboratory of Medical Biochemistry.

In the summer of 1986, Bruce Beutler left The Rockefeller University to become assistant investigator at the Howard Hughes Medical Institute in Dallas, Texas. His three years in the Laboratory of Medical Biochemistry had been prodigious, and in a letter on June 16, 1986, to Dr. Stephanie Vogel, at the F. Edward School of Medicine, he wrote that when in Dallas, he would "continue to study cachectin and related topics." Indeed, Bruce Beutler and Cerami continued to publish together on tumor necrosis, anemia, inflammation, cachectin, and shock until 1990.[47]

During this period, the controversy surrounding the potentially dangerous "dark side" of TNF began to recede as more laboratories were able to replicate the experimental findings that had been coming out of Cerami's lab. In the autumn of 1986, Kevin Tracey and the team began a series of experiments with an anti-TNF monoclonal antibody that specifically bound to TNF, neutralizing its toxicity.[48] Previous experiments on rodents were now superseded by an animal model of septic shock in baboons, which are anatomically and physiologically more similar to humans. Under Tracey's supervision, two anaesthetized baboons were placed side by side, catheters were then positioned in the femoral arteries, and the animals were placed under observation in conditions identical to that of an intensive care unit. The microbes selected for the experiment were a strain of bacteria isolated from a patient with septic shock. The researchers knew that injecting live bacteria would cause the baboons to develop septic shock,[49] but they did not know what would happen if they blocked it with antibodies. Accordingly, one of the infected animals was treated with the anti-TNF, which specifically inactivated the baboon's TNF by binding to it and rendering it invisible to the animal's tissues.[50] The other baboon received a different antibody that did not bind to TNF; subsequently, both animals were infused with a lethal dose of live bacteria. Within a few hours, the differences between the baboons' responses were, according to Tracey, "as dramatic as they were profound."[51] In both animals, TNF levels increased rapidly, but whereas the unprotected baboon developed shock and died within eight hours, the baboon treated with the anti-TNF monoclonal antibody was completely protected. Cerami "had never seen anything like it before"; the baboon had been given a massive amount of Escherichia coli but seemed completely unaffected. Within 24 hours, the animal resumed eating and living a normal life. Overjoyed at the results of their experimental breakthrough, many of the researchers stayed in the operating theater of the Cornell Medical School until 3 A.M. enjoying what Tracey described as "an incredible eureka moment, one of those elusive and memorable events that occurs, at best, only occasionally in a scientific career."[52] From their careful repeat experiments in baboons, the researchers showed that, for the best effects, antibodies needed to be administered two hours before the bacterial infusion. Now, more than ever, the team was convinced that it was TNF and not the bacteria that caused lethal septic shock. In December 1987, they published their results in Nature,[53] the impact of which completely metamorphosed the role of the molecule in disease causation and set in train a revolutionary redirection of the pharmaceutical industry. "These results," the article announced, "indicate that cachectin is a mediator of fatal bacteremic shock, and suggest that antibodies against cachectin offer a potential therapy of life-threatening protection."[54] By this time, both The Rockefeller University and Cornell Research Foundation Inc. had established an exclusive relationship with the Chiron Corporation, a biotechnology company in California. On November 12, in a letter to the company chairman William J. Rutter, Cerami wrote with understandable concern about the need to accelerate his laboratory's research on cachectin/TNF and his anxiety about where the bottlenecks lay: "we are in dire need of purified cachectin and neutralising antibodies."[55] Propitiously, through a collaborative interchange of scientists with The Rockefeller University, Chiron succeeded in providing the monoclonal antibody for the baboon experiment. The paper published in Nature has come to occupy the status of a classic in the medical canon, as it was the first ever therapeutic trial of a monoclonal antibody against TNF,[56] and the implications of this breakthrough reverberated throughout the biomedical world.

Cerami's curiosity and imagination that had led him to postulate—while sitting in cow manure in a Kenyan corral—that a molecule produced by the immune system was responsible for a variety of diseases contributed to a new era in medicine:

the cytokine theory of disease. This was discovery science at its finest, because for Cerami, who was driven by the desire to help patients, translational medicine was about connecting together discoveries in basic science to therapeutic end points. Not only did the cytokine theory of disease explain the causes of some chronic and acute diseases in patients, but crucially it also offered a variety of possible targets for monoclonal antibodies, a therapy that today accounts for a third of all new treatments.

In this spirit, the anti-TNF innovation was a necessary constituent of a wider scientific chain reaction that can be traced back to Rodney Porter's[57] work on antibodies, Cesar Milstein and Georges Kohler's discovery of monoclonal antibodies, and Richard Lerner and Greg Winter's mechanism to "humanize" monoclonal antibodies. As was noted earlier, infection is an important driver of evolution, and there are many aspects of our body's defense against invaders, viruses, and bacteria. One of the most important is by antibodies, protein molecules that are produced by B lymphocytes, a type of white blood cell crucial in protecting us against microbes. Antibodies are remarkable molecules because they are tailor-made so precisely that each individual antibody is directed to only one determinant—often a molecule specific to a microbe.[58] This diversity is mainly achieved through a process of cutting and pasting back together a vast number of small gene fragments in the developing B lymphocyte. In 1977, Georges Kohler and Cesar Milstein at the MRC Laboratory of Molecular Biology (LMB) in Cambridge (United Kingdom), an institution that famously had a Nobel laureate on every floor, were the first to make monoclonal antibodies (Mabs) by fusing B cells, making an antibody with a tumor cell, which provided limitless growth potential, to form a "hybridoma," a cell comprising genes from both cells and with properties of both. Each hybridoma made only one antibody, hence the term *monoclonal antibody*. Importantly, these are cancer cells that can be grown in huge number, providing virtually limitless quantities of antibody, with all molecules being essentially the same.

Between 1975 and 1986, when much of this innovative work was taking place, the biologist Sydney Brenner was director of the LMB in Cambridge. Partly out of annoyance at the large number of escaped fruit flies that inhabited the LMB's corridors, Brenner thought that the transparent nematode worm *Caenorhabditis elegans* would be a good model organism for the investigation of animal development—*C. elegans* subsequently became the first animal to have its complete genome sequenced. For this investigation of development biology, Brenner shared the Nobel Prize in Physiology or Medicine in 2002.[59] Brenner was known for his scientific genius and acerbic wit, both of which were demonstrated in his regular column "Loose Ends" in the journal *Current Biology*. I experienced Brenner's sense of humor firsthand in 2013 when I visited him in Ely, Cambridgeshire, where he was recuperating from a serious operation. "I'm feeling a lot better now," Brenner announced, "but I went into hospital with a colon, and came out with a semicolon." Brenner's discordant wit is also associated with the reporting of one of the LMB's greatest contributions to therapeutic medicine, the discovery of monoclonal antibodies. At one of the LMB's regular internal seminar meetings, which Brenner chaired, Cesar Milstein, the Argentinian-born biochemist and codiscoverer of monoclonal antibodies, was giving a talk on the possible applications of his invention.[60] Science, at least at the reporting stage, is a performance art, and unfortunately Milstein was not a compelling raconteur. But just before Brenner's concentration started to wander, it began to crystallize in his mind just what a profound discovery was being described: the invention of a method of forcing immune system cells to make pure antibodies against any chosen agent. Brenner immediately straightened up, and when the seminar ended, he asked Milstein, "Does this mean that theoretically, you could make an antibody against anything?" Looking around the room, Cesar Milstein tentatively answered, "Yes." Famously, Brenner quipped, "Could you make an antibody against my mother-in-law?"[61]

Cerami, with others, had shown how immune responses could be harmful to the host and that TNF could cause an acute shock syndrome during infections. Guided by these findings, the race was now on within the biotechnology sector to see if blocking TNF would be an effective treatment in patients with sepsis and septic shock. In the forefront of this research was the U.S. company Centocor, which had begun operations in 1979 by developing products based on monoclonal antibody technology. In 1986, Centocor launched Centoxin, a human antibody for the treatment of sepsis resulting from Gram-negative bacterial infection. The difficulty for Centocor or indeed any biotechnology company was the mechanism of the disease. As Kevin Tracey had discovered, TNF is produced so suddenly in cases of septic shock and acts so quickly to cause tissue injury that antibodies "would have to be given either before bacteria appeared on the scene, or within the first few minutes afterward."[62] Timing of treatment was a big issue,[63] and unless treatment was given before onset of the attack cascade, it had proved impossible to protect the patient from organ damage. As Kevin Tracey later wrote, without a medical crystal ball to predict future episodes of infection or septic shock, "we were stymied in our ability to treat patients . . . because their TNF peak would occur without warning."[64] Cerami's original idea, celebrated in his 1981 patent, was to make an antibody against rheumatoid arthritis, but because sepsis was such a big killer and the animal data so compelling, he became a leading advocate for the use of antibodies against the disease.[65] Nonetheless, the problem for pharmaceutical companies, and more importantly for patients, was that animal models did not accurately reflect the complex mechanism of the disease in humans.[66] Consequently, the optimism that had fueled the spending of tens of millions of dollars to find a monoclonal anti-TNF for use in severe infection came to an end after a series of clinical trial failures in the 1990s.[67] Centoxin had been in the vanguard of these experiments, but when the drug failed to establish indisputable efficacy, Centocor found itself in a financially difficult position, and its stock dropped from a high of $60 per share in December 1991 to $6 by April 1992. Despite the best efforts of translational scientists and leading pharmaceutical companies over the past twenty-five years, sepsis remains a leading cause of death in the United States.

A friend and colleague of Tony Cerami from the world of discovery science is Charles Dinarello, a clinical scientist widely considered one of the founding fathers of cytokines, having purified and cloned IL-1 and made the first IL-1 antibody. Cerami and Dinarello first met in 1981, at a National Institutes of Health conference, to discuss whether "TNF and IL-1 are the same molecule."[68] They are not, but they do the same thing; they both cause inflammation. Following that initial meeting, both men expanded the field of cytokine research in a way that helped to alter the therapeutic landscape. Cerami's laboratory had validated the concept that when the body is injured or invaded, TNF is the first cytokine to appear in the blood and that other proinflammatory mediators subsequently appear as part of an immunological cascade. But what was unknown at the time was whether Dinarello's IL-1 and another cytokine, IL-6, depended on TNF for their release into the bloodstream. This immunological mystery was answered unequivocally in 1989 by Cerami's lab in a paper published in the *Journal of Experimental Medicine*.[69] Yuman Fong, a surgeon at Cornell Medical Center, was first author on the paper, which suggested that "cachectin/TNF is essential for the initiation or amplification of IL-1 and IL-6 release during lethal gram-negative septic shock syndrome." Although the paper is not the most cited of the early cachectin/TNF investigations, thirty years after its publication, Fong looks upon the article as the most important research finding of his scientific studies undertaken in Cerami's lab. "The work was a huge group effort and we showed that by blocking TNF you didn't see the firing of either IL-1 or IL-6, and that just blocking one step can actually modulate an entire pathway."[70] This discovery highlighted the importance of TNF in the pathogenesis of inflammatory disorders and provided further evidence that the molecule would be a good target for anticytokine therapy.

Charles Dinarello maintains his reputation in the scientific community as a major interlocutor in cytokine history. His name is not merely associated with IL-1; it metaphorically inhabits the molecule. To reinforce his association with the molecule, he has T-shirts made for his colleagues and even wears a baseball cap emblazoned with the moniker "IL-1 beta"; he is, in effect, Mr. IL-1. After twenty years of sticking thermometers in the rear end of rabbits and successfully making the first cytokine antibody in 1977, Charles Dinarello has made a scientific contribution that has endured. Dinarello's scientific career and renown has, in many respects, been defined over the past half century by IL-1; he has stayed with the inflammatory molecule, never strayed and never left. But there was no such adhesion for Tony Cerami to TNF; instead of staying and making the molecule eternally synonymous with his science, he effectively, according to Dinarello, "dropped out of TNF."[71] Between 1995 and 2010, Tony Cerami published only two papers directly related to TNF, which may have contributed to obscuring his original and indispensable contribution to understanding the protein's biological function. Undoubtedly, one of Cerami's great abilities was to harness his curiosity of the natural world and conduct basic research with the aim of developing drugs for use in the clinic. In this respect, Cerami was the quintessential translational scientist and a leading proponent of rational drug discovery, but, as Dinarello recognizes, even for Cerami, defining therapeutic targets and making the jump from animal models in the laboratory to use in patients in the clinic is a biologically complex undertaking with little chance of success: "the antibody unfortunately didn't work in shock. If the antibody had worked in septic shock Tony would be very famous today. I sometimes tell my students, 'don't get involved in shock, it's a cemetery for good molecules.'"[72]

Even after the failure with sepsis, Cerami was widely regarded as a gifted scientist,[73] and what set him apart from many of his contemporaries was the extraordinary diversity of his interests. Not content with one or two ideas to pursue over a career, Cerami determinedly followed half a dozen research ideas simultaneously. In a positive sense, the enviable span of interest was made possible by his innate boundary-hopping mode of cognition, and the broad horizon perspective he practiced created what is termed nowadays as "elastic thinking," enabling new ideas to materialize in moments of insight. But he could also be capricious. Like many scientists, he found research addictive. The cosmic thinking that set the early trajectory of a research path toward making a new discovery, the heightening of the senses, and the excitement that flowed at the thought of being able to see something for the first time were sometimes irresistible. This scientific existentialism, which drove Cerami, was noted by his daughter Carla: "he pushes things forward [and] he always goes his own way, my dad."[74] Just like Martin Arrowsmith in Sinclair Lewis's eponymous novel, Cerami is an idealist, his aim being to use science to unlock the mysteries and ills of the human body. Cerami, occupying a location at the frontiers of biomedical research, was in a privileged position that, by its very nature, offered tempting new destinations, especially if the ground being currently occupied had become complicated either personally or scientifically. And there was a perception that the failure of TNF blockade in sepsis did take a toll on Cerami.[75] However, being enthralled by the allure of the new can also act as a distraction and erode the historical contribution made by long-standing research programs. As a consequence, one of the scientific criticisms of Cerami was that rarely was something pursued in depth,[76] that his forte was the wide breadth of knowledge that pulled together ideas from different fields that gave a unique perspective on the mechanisms of whatever disease he wanted his lab to work on. But once some level of success had been achieved, his focus invariably moved onto the next disease. One of the many important discoveries made by Cerami's lab was identifying TNF's association with a multiplicity of illnesses ranging from parasitic diseases[77] to those associated with chronic inflammation.[78] Indeed, the failure of monoclonal antibodies to arrest the progress of sepsis in humans did not lead to a diminution of interest in this new therapeutic pathway— far from it, in fact. Rather, it acted as a catalyst to other dedicated and highly motivated researchers to enter the anti-TNF field.

Today, it may well seem unthinkable, even inconceivable, but when the history of the therapeutic and commercial success of anti-TNF is being considered, Tony

Cerami's name may not feature as prominently as either he or his supporters think justified. This is in part explained by a discernible leitmotif in the scientific career of Tony Cerami in which disagreements, conflicts of ego, and the who, what, when, and where of discovery have led to abrupt shifts of direction sometimes so galvanic that they could be interpreted almost as acts of self-sabotage. As we shall see, not all of the personal and scientific redirections and ruptures were planned or designed because, as Soren Kierkegaard, the first existential philosopher, noted, "Life has to be lived forward, but it can only be understood backward."[79] Certainly, one causal factor for Cerami's relative anonymity in the TNF story is that he may have failed to contribute sufficiently to the scientific literature, and as his friend Charles Dinarello freely admits, "Writing is not his priority, he doesn't want to blow his own horn—I get that. I tend to blow my own horn, I'm proud of what I did. But he is not as well known for his discoveries as he should be. The clinicians get all of the credit for anti-TNF, but Tony left TNF and went into chemokins. When you ask people today about TNF they don't say 'Tony Cerami.'"[80]

On occasion, during the long labor-intensive route of drug discovery, the basic science element in a successful pharmaceutical story can become overshadowed when the drug is brought to final testing and shown to be efficacious. Of course, this is not the outcome of a deliberate conspiracy or something that would conform to the British epidemiologist Bradford Hill's "criteria for causation," but frequently the individuals who are the final link in the scientific chain from conception to successful therapeutic receive a disproportionate share of the limelight compared to those scientists who made the original breakthrough. Who, for instance, will recall the contribution of the inimitable biochemist, Norman Heatley, to the therapeutic discovery of penicillin in Oxford in the 1940s? Alexander Fleming, Howard Florey, and Ernst Chain shared the 1945 Nobel Prize in Physiology or Medicine "for the discovery of penicillin and its curative effects in various infectious diseases,"[81] but it was Heatley who, with dexterous skills and practical mind, constructed the futuristic apparatus that produced the elusive antibiotic that revolutionized biomedical science. Much indeed can be lost by the time the drug arrives in the clinic—and good science is often polarizing.

9 · LEAVING THE ROCKEFELLER UNIVERSITY
The End of the Dream

If I know myself, I work from a sort of instinct to try to make out truth.
—Charles Darwin

The decade of the 1980s marked the pinnacle of Cerami's scientific career at The Rockefeller University. During that decisive period, he became a powerful figure, influencing the direction of science at his beloved institution; joined the editorial board of the highly influential *Journal of Experimental Medicine*; was appointed dean of graduate and postgraduate studies; won several prestigious prizes; and employed large numbers of researchers across a variety of biomedical subjects. His elevation in the scientific hierarchy was reflected figuratively in the new location of the Laboratory of Medical Biochemistry. From the C Floor bottom basement in Theobald Smith Hall, it metamorphosed into occupying the entire sixteenth floor of the Tower, a new high-tech edifice of biomedical modernity. Situated on the building's penultimate floor, immediately below the dining hall, the lab and Cerami's office provided an enviable panoramic view over the East River. Inhabiting such an illustrious position in the aristocracy of scientific research, one could be forgiven for thinking that Cerami may have felt a sense of personal and professional satisfaction. After all, he was, and remains, the only former Rockefeller graduate student to become the dean of The Rockefeller University. He had worked his way up through the ranks of a Darwinian cutthroat environment to reach the highest echelons of academic science, and yet, he recognized that there were residual scientific tensions at play within the intellectual fabric of the university. It was to be these divergent views about the future financing, direction, and organization of academic science at The Rockefeller University that culminated in a period of what one historian described as "internal turmoil"[1] at the beginning of the 1990s that dramatically affected the course of Cerami's life.

Compared to the straitened circumstances in which he lived as a child on the family's poultry farm[2] in rural New Jersey, he now lived a charmed life[3] exemplified by the respect in which he was held within the scientific community and by

the trappings of growing affluence. Cerami never entirely broke free of his impecunious past and was held captive by its distant grasp; he knew only too well what it
was like to suffer economic hardship, saw no virtue in poverty, and was determined
never to be poor again. A measure of just how quickly Cerami broke free, at least
materially, from his background to ascend the social class pyramid can be gleaned
from an internal letter that he wrote on December 29, 1982, to Mr. Zachary J. Contes
of The Rockefeller University: "Dear Jack, We would like to change our apartment
with respect to the kitchen and the mall terrace. Our recent decision to build a
summer house on Shelter Island confirms our staying in our present apartment and necessitates the modification."[4] The rapid transition from rural priva-
tion to commissioning an architect-designed home adjacent to the highly desirable
shores of Long Island, for generations the preserve of New York's wealthy and
artistic elites, was further evidence of Cerami's growing wealth and status. By the
end of the 1980s, the social transformation from hardscrabble beginnings to wield-
ing considerable power within the scientific establishment was completed when
Cerami moved his family from Rockefeller accommodation into an apartment on
Park Avenue.

Over the preceding years, Cerami had succeeded in creating a special atmosphere in the lab through his charismatic personality[5] and youthful enthusiasm. His
aim was to replicate the atmosphere that he had experienced as a graduate student
over twenty years earlier, when the feeling was that at The Rockefeller University,
the sky was the limit. It was a place where students were allowed the freedom to
think for themselves and encouraged to think big. Above all, Cerami wanted
researchers to enjoy and revel in science,[6] to bounce ideas off each other, to excite
each other, and to feel free and protected. He was justifiably proud of his MD/PhD
students and their ability to break new ground, to be kaleidoscopic in their interests as well as accomplished experimentalists at the bench. During the summer of
1980, one of those students, Peter Hotez, joined the laboratory and found Cerami's scientific philosophy, with its focus on the disease rather than a particular
field of scientific inquiry, captivating. For a young researcher like Hotez, early
exposure to the forces of encouragement is never forgotten: "I remember how
generous Tony was with his time, often meeting me for breakfast in the cafeteria to
kick around new ideas for a doctoral dissertation."[7] Ideas have consequences, and
it was in Cerami's lab that Hotez learned how to apply a knowledge of chemistry
to understand the mechanisms of parasitical diseases and develop drugs to treat
them. Cerami's outstanding ability was to choose talent, and importantly, he could
nurture talent. More of a mentor than a manager, his lasting contribution was his
downstream influence on generations of productive translational scientists.

It was Cerami's ability to relate to young graduate students that drew the attention of President Joshua Lederberg, the Board of Trustees, and Chairman David
Rockefeller when a new dean of graduate and postgraduate studies was required
in 1986, after the departure of virologist Purnell W. Choppin. Cerami's appointment was uncontentious as he was liked by his peers and he knew the Rockefeller

family well, having even taken their grandchildren on tours of the animal facility and labs on a number of occasions. But, for his own part, there was one stipulation: he would only take on the role of dean if his colleague, Miki Rifkin, was retained in her position of associate dean. Indeed, during subsequent years, as Cerami's scientific power and responsibilities expanded exponentially in the outside world, no one doubted that the *real* dean was Miki Rifkin, who effectively ran the graduate school and maintained the academic-political equipoise via a combination of genuinely enjoying the company of students and knowing the arcana of institutional procedures and the judicious use of power. But Cerami was no mere figurehead; he felt an overwhelming loyalty and sense of indebtedness to that great vintage of scientists, including Peyton Rous, George Palade, and Detlev Bronk, who had instilled in him a sense of belonging. Now, in his turn, he wanted to use the office of dean to make the student body feel justly indispensable. Some of his methods, it must be said, were more unconventional than others. By way of injecting some life into the underused faculty club and encouraging scientific conversations and mentorship, Cerami decided on a very antiprohibitionist policy of free beer, which was bought at $50 a case and distributed among the students when they visited the faculty bar. "So, I went ahead," the moderate-drinking Cerami remembered, "and bought the beer and invited the students to come to the club between 4 and 6 P.M., I figured that the students would stay on when the junior faculty came in. Strangely, everybody felt good about the innovation except the faculty." Perhaps this was because they were the only ones paying for drinks!

Another early initiative was his campaign to raise money among faculty to buy a small fleet of secondhand vans that students could borrow free of charge. At the time, a driver had to be twenty-five to rent a car in New York, which effectively disqualified most of the student body, so being able to have the freedom to escape the city for a freewheeling weekend break was liberating. The plan was simple: the vans were free to use, but students were responsible for maintaining them in good working order. Cerami also sponsored organized picnics, which gave the students access to faculty members and opened up opportunities to exchange ideas and to do something that Cerami believed to be of profound importance and of lasting value—mentorship. Similarly, programs were put in place to encourage students to try activities that they would not normally have the opportunity to do. In this vein, he accompanied groups to piano recitals on the famous floating barge moored in Brooklyn and even secured a box at the Metropolitan Opera—to expose students to aspects of culture that had been absent from his own background. Of course, he was still the dean, and regardless of how outwardly benevolent Cerami behaved toward the students, it must nevertheless have been a daunting experience for prospective biochemists attending an interview for a place at The Rockefeller University to be asked to draw the structure of glucose or ATP on the blackboard in his office.[8]

While no one could accuse Cerami of having an inferiority complex, there was no denying that when he first arrived in New York City in the early 1960s, he was conscious that some of his contemporaries, especially those from Ivy League schools and other private universities, possessed a conversational ease and knowledge of the arts that had been lacking in his education thus far. He too wanted to know more about Mary McCarthy's latest novel—*The Group* appeared in 1963, the year after his arrival at the The Rockefeller University—or critique a stanza from a poem by Robert Frost or Langston Hughes. So profound was his determination to make good this deficiency that very early on, he made a promise to himself to read a book of fiction, poetry, or drama every week over the five years of his PhD. In truth, when he arrived at the Rockefeller, he did not feel particularly "polished," but neither did he feel "unpolished"; it was just that he felt an overwhelming compulsion to broaden his cultural canvas. This was another example of the "self-help" spirit that was instilled in childhood. Nonetheless, the central and overwhelming message coming from the dean's office during those years was that science was the way forward and that "science is fun."[9] But Cerami was also serious in his efforts to try to lessen the demarcation lines between science and the humanities, as well as provide ways for students to experience greater emotional enrichment and a broader human perspective. Primarily, Cerami recognized that biomedical education did not always fully prepare graduate students to recognize and respond appropriately to all the facets of human nature they would encounter in later professional life. What does is good literature, and the emotional literacy and honest self-appraisal that can be gained from reading Leo Tolstoy, Philip Roth, and Sylvia Plath was an objective that Cerami sought to promote both in his own life and in the lives of others. To Cerami's mind, an appreciation of the fragile interconnectedness of disciplines such as science, history, and literature taught all of us how to see more clearly and understand the world around us more fully. This was in part because he was only too aware of how human frailty drove historical events and that while he could list the great advances that had been made in medical science,[10] he was also mindful that the forces of displacement and dispossession would be constant themes shaping the future.

Paralleling his work as dean, Cerami's commitment to biomedical science accelerated as the decade of the 1980s progressed, and to carry out truly effective research requires a detailed plan together with some other essential components. In the opinion of the German immunologist Paul Ehrlich, successful scientific work required the four Gs: *geschick* (skill), *geluld* (patience), *geld* (money), and *gluck* (luck).[11] Cerami greatly admired Ehrlich's scientific attitude. Unfortunately, Ehrlich did not explain how to acquire the last of these essential requirements, but Cerami was clear in his own mind that good luck, or serendipity, was probably more likely to play a role if skill, patience, and a rigorous program of experimentation had been followed. He was also particularly intolerant of researchers who contravened his ideal of what it was to be an effective translational scientist, that is, to make products for use in the clinic and not merely a dedication to securing the next National Institutes of Health (NIH) grant.[12] At one time during the 1980s, Cerami employed over fifty scientists in his lab, and he could be an uncompromising taskmaster, holding particular opprobrium for researcher workers who had a negative attitude. This was demonstrated memorably to one postdoc who had been given N1 Alpha (interferon alpha-n1) to work on and, even though he was a very good scientist, had made no progress on the project whatsoever. Surgeon Yuman Fong happened to be attending one of the regular lab meetings on the day that Cerami's patience finally ran out: "Tony said to the postdoc, 'You're fired. Because for a year, every day you've come in and thought of reasons why not to do experiments, I need people who come in every day and think of reasons to do experiments and make advances!' This reproach made an enormous impact on me and I've said it a lot of times over the past thirty years that people should come to work thinking of experiments that they need to do, not the other way round. It stuck with me, and Tony's thinking has been enormously important in my life."[13] Cerami pursued NIH money and garnered NIH support, but what was sacrosanct was discovery science. "Following the science" was the mantra of his laboratory.

This was a time when Cerami and his team felt completely unrestrained by boundaries: they did not limit their investigations to orphan diseases, parasitology, diabetology, or protein modifications of disease; they were constantly searching to find new treatments and, if at all possible, to have some fun while doing it. Cerami too was conscious that in translational medicine, making a discovery is a completely random occurrence, but what was important was to ask the right questions: how do we treat and diagnose disease, and what can we usefully learn from understanding basic mechanisms in the human body to provide useful knowledge that can help people? Fail or succeed, and adjust accordingly—that was the philosophy. The search for better solutions to health is, as it should be, ceaseless.

One notable success, made in 1985, was the discovery of the mechanism of action of arsenical drugs in the treatment of trypanosomiasis. British physician-scientist Alan Fairlamb, who joined the lab in 1981, was asked by Cerami to find a missing enzyme from trypanosomes that enabled the parasites to fend off free radicals produced by the immune system of the host. After eighteen grueling months of hard work, Fairlamb finally discovered a unique dithiol found only in African parasites that he named *trypanothione*, which was an enzyme of central importance as an intracellular protectant. The parasitology group then published its findings,[14] which marked a period of great excitement in the lab because not only did it offer suggestions of the how arsenical and antitrypanosomal agents worked, but also it signposted a new dimension for direct discovery.

Ironically, the sheer diversity of Cerami's interests, together with his originality and ubiquity in the scientific literature, brought an extraordinary admonishment from the nation's leading scientific institution that most scientists could only dream of receiving. In 1987, after being site visited by the NIH, Cerami burst into Alan Fairlamb's office enraged at what had just happened. "Can you believe it," Cerami bellowed in disbelief, "I've just been criticized by someone on the NIH committee for publishing too much in *Science* and *Nature*!"[15] After a moment's reflection, Fairlamb replied, "Tony, they might have a point there."[16] Fairlamb's exoneration of the NIH's censure is partly explained by the belief that publishing an article in *Science* or *Nature* was seen as putting down a marker on a particular field and that conventionally, the article would then be followed up with the detailed under-pinnings of the broad brush strokes in a specialty journal. Undeniably, the views of the NIH fed into a judgment, held by others, that not enough of Cerami's scien-tific research had been followed up in sufficient depth.[17] But this criticism also raises two fundamental questions—what defines the scientific method, and what is the embodiment of the scientific mind? Is it the spark of insight and imagina-tion that should be lionized and cultivated, or is it the careful methodological approach that more generally leads to scientific enlightenment and progress? What-ever the thinking, Cerami was very much the quintessence of the former, with his voracious curiosity and imagination[18] allied to the ability to see patterns and to propagate theories. It did not matter particularly whether those theories turned out to be true or not because by the time a hypothesis was going to be tested, Cerami may have moved on to generate new hypotheses in other areas. Cerami's strength as a scientist was that he was a trailblazer ahead of his time[19] with the capacity to bring together different fields to give new insights into disease processes. The real-ity is that science needs the white heat of trailblazers just as much as it requires the methodological techniques of the careful systematic scientist. What is important to recognize is that both approaches characterize aspects of the scientific mind and are both equally indispensable. Over a period of three decades, one feature of Cerami's work was incontestable: nothing he did was far removed from some human disease. And as he walked across the expanse of his lab, with the critique of the NIH still reverberating in his mind, he felt emotionally conflicted between confusion and understandable redemption, because from the very beginning, like many other scientists, his ambition was to publish his ideas in *Science* and *Nature*.

Throughout his life in translational medicine, Cerami's successes were punctu-ated by myriad failures and years of disillusionment at the bench.[20] What kept him going was the excitement of discovery, the camaraderie of the lab, and knowl-edge that occasionally along the way, a discovery might lead to some lasting good for humanity. At its best, the Laboratory of Medical Biochemistry was formidably productive and a formative center of scientific investigation that exposed its mem-bers to a unique scientific culture that encouraged dedication, honesty, and cour-age. In Cerami's mind, there is an underlying humanity to pursuing science; he sees it as a noble endeavor that demands intellectual rigor, persistence, devotion, and considerable sacrifice to produce even the most rudimentary insights into the law of nature. From the origin of the scientific method dating from Francis Bacon in the seventeenth century, profound visionaries like Faraday and outstanding experimental innovators like Koch and Ehrlich had sought to understand the bio-logical *mechanisms* that lay at the heart of human illness. Other investigators saw science as primarily ignorance driven, involving the comprehensive collection of data, which then provides a resource for others to test their own hypotheses. Con-versely, Cerami sought to understand disease mechanisms by synthesizing the skills of biologists, biochemists, parasitologists, and organic chemists to discover better treatments for neglected, orphan, and noncommunicable diseases. A special scientific alchemy was created in the lab, and for many of those who worked there in the 1980s, the experience was transformative, shaping the thinking of the next generation of applied scientists.[21] This attitude encapsulated perhaps the oldest pedagogical system known—the apprentice system: a tried and tested relationship whereby promising young researchers learn by assisting senior scientists at work.[22] There was a conscious focus on making therapies to benefit the human race in a tangible therapeutic way, with Cerami playing more the role of a mentor than a manager. In 2006, Alan Fairlamb and Mike Ferguson, another Rockefeller researcher who worked in George Cross's lab, established the interdisciplinary Drug Discovery Unit in Dundee, Scotland, which today is home to one of the world's leading parasitology units developing new medicines for malaria, trypanosomiasis, and other neglected tropical diseases.

Of course, in addition to the sacrifices and achievements of a life in science, there are important elements that have a value metric beyond the discoveries made in the lab or contributions to the published literature, however brilliant, insightful, or influential. To cell biologist Daniel Rifkin, who still has a lab at NYU and is a friend and contemporary of Tony Cerami, there are essentially only two lasting things that can be taken from a life spent in science. "One is your enjoyment that comes from doing the science, and the other is the sense of satisfaction you get from the people that you train. Everything else, once you stop, it's gone. Nobody refers to your work, and how many Francis Cricks are there? Few."[23] By these criteria, Cerami certainly did have a fulfilling career at The Rockefeller University. He loved the institution, and among the many recognized scientific accomplishments and disappointments, there was also much excitement, discovery, and fun. Cerami was also capable of being a terrific mentor, showing unbending loyalty and dedication to many of the young men and women who came within his scientific orbit. But Cerami was not always a benign presence; his creativity was driven by ambition, and some relationships became complicated due in part to his mercurial personality and equally to the inherent tensions flowing through his scientific and personal life, which were at times enthrallingly and complicatedly interwoven. In common with many people, Cerami is a character of intense contradictions and more complicated than he appears; he can be a good friend and a fine role model for how one should approach research and discovery science, but also, on occasion, he could be difficult to work with. Even those he was very close to could be cold-shouldered or given the "silent treatment"[24]; others stopped working with him under circumstances that were not pleasant, and while they left the lab as friends, they perceived a potential for losing the friendship if they had stayed. These were the uncomfortable truths, the by-products of the cut and thrust of discovery science with all of its accompanying interpersonal and financial pressures. They were bruising encounters far removed from the in-house disparagements that Howard Florey would regularly deliver to the young researchers who populated his laboratory in Oxford. Rather than looking back on some withering remark with affection as a piece of much treasured Floriana,[25] for those in Cerami's group who felt the chill wind of ostracism, they were forever marked by the rejection. If Cerami's personality was a contributing factor in some of these intermittent tensions with his team, an infinitely more complex and delicately layered relationship existed with his wife and scientific colleague, Helen Vlassara. Increasingly, as Helen's career blossomed, there was a corresponding shift in the internal dynamics of their life together; from being a scientific mentor offering guidance and leadership, Cerami felt the bilateral intruding presence of steely competition. This polarizing force would not only bring an end to their scientific partnership, which for two decades had helped to define and consolidate the field of AGEs, but it would also contribute to the breakup of their marriage.

Within the tempo of flux and stasis, one constant in the administration of all things scientific in the Laboratory of Medical Biochemistry was the guiding presence of Kirk Manogue. From the outset of his career at the Rockefeller, Cerami liked to work in tandem with someone he could trust and, better still, an intellectual equal and a sane arbitrator of which research programs might provide the best prospects of success. For more than a decade, Kirk Manogue was the custodian of the lab's multifarious research programs, providing an invaluable scientific buffer zone that allowed his boss to be free from the daily minutia of lab administration and to concentrate on the cosmic thinking that underpinned the culture of translational medicine. But Manogue was much more than a scientific administrator; he was a brilliant graduate of The Rockefeller University. In addition to being a gifted judge of talent, he was erudite and, according to one scientist, "Kirk was Tony's amminus, he was a very good writer who could focus on the detail of grant applications and patents, skills that Tony needed, and he was also very close to what was going on in the lab at the bench."[26] Cerami looked upon Manogue as his friend, closest confidante, "another arm, my protector, my lawyer," and, in a linguistic allusion to his Sicilian heritage, "my consigliere." Because of the importance of this professional relationship, Cerami was adamant that he would never embark upon a new scientific project without the inimitable support from his most reliable and principled colleague.

In the spring of 1987, Kenneth Warren's noble efforts to introduce biomedical science to the study of infectious diseases was interrupted when he was unceremoniously stripped of his power and eased out of the Rockefeller Foundation. The conclusion of the landmark ten-year Great Neglected Diseases of Mankind Program (GND) was marked by a final scientific meeting held under the snows of Mt. Kilimanjaro, at the Taita Hills Wildlife Sanctuary, Kenya. From its inception, each year the GND meetings became bigger, more rambunctious, and scientifically memorable. Close friendships were established between many outstanding researchers, and the annual event became rather more like a reunion or perhaps a family gathering. Cerami assiduously attended every meeting and always brought with him a varied cohort of the brightest and best from his lab who were dedicated to finding new treatments for ancient scourges. This was the embodiment of the ideal envisaged by the GND, and the flexibility of the financial support that Warren offered enabled Cerami and other researchers to develop overseas links and to carry out fieldwork that would have otherwise been impossible.[27]

To the final meeting, Cerami brought with him two parasitologists, together with the translational scientist Barbara Sherry and his young son Ethan. Arriving some days before the meeting, Cerami hired a large 4 × 4 and took the group on a safari tour of the Rift Valley, staying in the isolated villages that he and his team of parasitologists had worked with over the course of the previous decade. It was the trip of a lifetime.[28] Barbara Sherry was one of a generation of scientists who owed her career to Cerami's tutelage and ability to nurture talent. In Sherry's case, the springboard to securing a firm foothold on the ladder of academic science came serendipitously. Cerami, who had a history of back problems, had been poleaxed by back pain and was incapacitated while on a lecture tour in California. The injury had a knock-on effect, coming as it did during a critical stage in the application process for funding, and unable to get back to New York City, Cerami instructed Sherry to apply for the NIH grant in his absence. The application proved successful, and its acquisition transformed Sherry's career in terms of self-confidence, prestige, and standing among her peers. After the days spent in the splendor of the Masai Mara Game Reserve, Cerami and his group joined the GND meeting, where Sherry gave her inaugural presentation expertly assisted by Ethan, who projected the slides that accompanied her talk.

The days spent in the Taita Hills were enormously productive, and although they came to represent the end of one historic experiment in the nascent field of what we know today as global health, the program inspirited other audacious projects that sought to focus the world's attention on infectious diseases. One notable example is the KEMRI Wellcome Trust Research Programme, which was established in 1989 in Kilifi on the east coast of Kenya. Its first director was British physician-scientist Kevin Marsh, who had a broad interest in the clinical, epidemiological, and immunological aspects of malaria and childhood diseases. Quite by chance, Marsh spent some time at the GND meeting in Taita Hills while he was traveling around Africa: "It was while I was attending the meeting in 1987, that I ended up going down to Kilifi . . . and the die was cast!"[29] Marsh spent over twenty-five years on the east coast of Kenya developing an interdisciplinary program addressing many aspects of public health in Africa.

The remarkable GND program lasted from 1978 to 1987, and during those years, Cerami and his group had made valuable contributions to the list of neglected tropical diseases that Warren had prioritized. The program was renowned for its collectivist character and the scientific impact of its collaborative efforts. There was much to celebrate, foremost among which was the deep bond of friendship between Warren and Cerami. The only note of unease for Cerami was the unexpected presence at the meeting of Nobel laureate David Baltimore. Cerami and Baltimore had been graduate students together at the Rockefeller in the 1960s, and they were not friends. Baltimore was at Taita Hills accompanying his wife, biologist Dr. Alice Huang, who was part of Warren's GND team. During the week-long conference, David Baltimore and Cerami scrupulously maintained a courteous relationship.

During the 1980s, there was a growing perception in the Laboratory of Medical Biochemistry that The Rockefeller University's historic interest in basic science and genetics was increasingly at odds with Cerami and other investigators' commitment to translational medicine. This cultural tension had frustrated Cerami since his early failed attempts to persuade the university's administrators to patent his measurement of HbA1c as a method of metabolic control. That failure had been a salutatory experience and disabused him of the belief that he could materially affect the growth of translational science within the university's wider scientific corpus.[30] By the end of the 1980s, both within and outside The Rockefeller University, there was a growing awareness that the institution was not performing as well as it had been in previous decades.[31] There were, it must be said, extenuating circumstances: the center of gravity of U.S. science was increasingly moving westward, and New York City was becoming prohibitively expensive for junior faculty. As a consequence, it became progressively more difficult for the university to recruit scientists of their first choice. The recruitment program was further hindered by accusations of oligarchic rule, that the university was organized as an agglomeration of scientific baronies, each under the control of a senior professor—a system that precluded few if any junior faculty from securing their own laboratories or achieving any semblance of autonomy in research.[32] This supposed stifling of scientific ambition was the exact antithesis of Cerami's career at The Rockefeller University. He had progressed rapidly up the phylogenetic tree of academic science, becoming a fully autonomous professor at the age of thirty-eight within the increasingly maligned Rockefeller system. He still felt closely connected to the scientific currents of late twentieth-century science and found the university a wonderfully creative environment in which to work, but during the presidency of Joshua Lederberg, problems began to appear, not least the realization that The Rockefeller University was no longer immune to fluctuations in the U.S. economy. Throughout the twentieth century, the two John D. Rockefellers were always available to allocate funds in times of financial stress, but the severity of the economic downturn led to the university imposing a salary freeze and running an annual deficit of $12 million.[33] With changes occurring at an ever-increasing rate in the larger world of science, the university became labeled as a paternalistic institution dominated by older scientists out of touch with the times scientifically and otherwise. By the end of the decade, what The Rockefeller University needed was a generation of Cerami-like scientists—men and women who were inhabiting emerging currents in biomedical research and who could quickly rise through the ranks of the scientific community. Instead, in 1989, the average age of tenured faculty was fifty-eight. Manifestly, the university had lost its sense of mission and was in urgent need of reform. To recapture its dominant influence over biomedical science,

David Rockefeller and the board of trustees decided that the presidency should be entrusted to an elite scientist who had earned his doctorate at The Rockefeller University and was also regarded as a successful administrator. Accordingly, in the autumn of 1989, it was announced that David Baltimore was going to succeed Joshua Lederberg as president of The Rockefeller University. Baltimore won the Nobel Prize in Physiology or Medicine in 1975 and had been known among biologists as a wunderkind for some time.[34] It was reported by one of his friends that the presidency of The Rockefeller University was Baltimore's "lifelong dream."[35] When Tony Cerami heard the news of Baltimore's appointment, he was heartbroken. "I went to see David Rockefeller and I told him that Baltimore's presidency was going to be a terrible idea and that it was going to cause turmoil. But it was a done deal— with no faculty input. I would have taken anybody except David Baltimore."[36]

David Baltimore's presidency not only formed a crucial episode in Cerami's life but also witnessed the stormiest two years in the Rockefeller's history and framed a troubling episode between the intimately interwoven worlds of science and politics in the United States. From the outset, Baltimore's appointment was strongly opposed by Cerami and other members of the senior faculty who had known Baltimore since their graduate student days together in the 1960s and intensely disliked his arrogance. To be sure, it was not only the past that they were worried about. Baltimore's appointment was vehemently resisted primarily because of the complex and unresolved controversy concerning a scientific paper that he and several of his Massachusetts Institute of Technology (MIT) collaborators had published in *Cell* in 1986.[37] The authenticity of what would have normally been an obscure and esoteric article became a scientific cause célèbre that snowballed into a visceral dispute about laboratory fraud that pitted Baltimore and his many supporters in the scientific community against Congress and Senator John D. Dingell's House Subcommittee on Oversight and Investigations.[38] The internecine five-year power struggle over alleged fake data became known as *The Baltimore Case*, the full story of which was eloquently described in Daniel J. Kevles's crisp, clear, and meticulously researched book in 1998.[39] The circumstances surrounding the case were not in dispute. In 1986, Baltimore and Dr. Thereza Imanishi-Kari of Tufts University and others published a research article in the journal *Cell*. After publication, Dr. Margot O'Toole, an untenured researcher at Tufts, told Dr. Imanishhi-Kari that she believed repeat measurements for the experiment had not been carried out. Dr. O'Toole then took the complaint to Baltimore, who dismissed her charges as, later, did an MIT panel (where David Baltimore was the director of the Whitehead Institute). Dr. O'Toole lost her job. The case was subsequently examined by two different NIH investigations, one of which exonerated Dr. Imanishi-Kari of faking data, while the other reported that the disputed data were indeed fabricated. The case generated more than a thousand pages of congressional testimony, hundreds of pages of comment, and extensive exchanges in *Nature* and elsewhere[40] that led to what *Time Magazine* described as an "icy confrontation"[41] in 1989 between Baltimore and Senator John Dingell. Throughout the dispute, David Baltimore consistently defended the integrity of his colleague, Dr. Imanishi-Kari.[42] Baltimore was never suspected of faking anything himself,[43] but his handling of the case and the media's coverage of the scientific community's ethics and practices brought unwanted attention to The Rockefeller University. The issues surrounding the *Cell* paper simply would not disappear, and in 1989, when Cerami was interviewed by a *New York Times* reporter, he said that Baltimore "actually helped precipitate the thing and make it worse for himself and science in general."[44] And Baltimore's handling of the case "got him in more trouble than if he had handled it in a straightforward manner from the beginning" and the apparent hubris was "a bellwether of his character."

From a purely professional standpoint, Cerami genuinely believed that Baltimore could not serve as president while contesting a protracted congressional investigation at the same time,[45] but from a personal point of view, he dearly hoped that the hearings in Washington—which were described in some quarters as a "witch hunt" and portrayed Dingell as a "new McCarthy"—would bring an end to the new president's tenure.[46] If the gloves were off in the public domain,[47] things were no better within the internal power politics of The Rockefeller University. More than a third of the senior faculty joined Cerami in openly declaring their heartfelt opposition to David Baltimore, including the Nobel laureate Gerald M. Edelman. Cerami and Edelman had never been allies before, but their mutual unhappiness with Baltimore united them in common cause. Having known Baltimore from graduate school days in the 1960s, Edelman devised an exit strategy and removed himself directly from the fray, later becoming a professor of neurobiology at the Scripps Research Institute in San Diego, California. Other leading dissenters who felt that Baltimore's presence would be detrimental to the institution's public image were Zanvil A. Cohn and Gunter Blobel. As dean of the university, and having the trust of senior faculty, Cerami became the nexus of communication between his colleagues and Baltimore. It was a deeply uncomfortable role for Cerami. However, there was a growing acceptance that Baltimore was, after all, going to be appointed president and that rather than resentment, everyone should be guided by the better angels of their nature, forsake the past, shake hands, and work in harmony for the collective good of the institution.

Accordingly, a "clear the air" meeting was scheduled for 2 P.M. on October 10, 1989. David Baltimore arrived late for the meeting with Cerami, Cohn, and Blobel, and far from coming in a spirit of appeasement, he was imperious and belligerent. Verbatim notes of the meeting taken by Cerami reveal the lingering schisms between the new president and the status quo.

> After a brief handshake D.B. in an aggressive and hostile tone and attitude began attacking the three of us. He began by stating that he had heard nothing from anyone or read in the papers anything that would dissuade him from taking the job. In fact, the article that appeared in the Times that morning made it impossible for

him not to take the position. He then accused us of saying that he was guilty of misdoing when he was not in fact.

We assured him that this was not what we said but neither (*sic*) we felt that his handling of the affair at the beginning did not show maturity or leadership abilities. With complete confidence he reclaimed that he had the ability and backing of the board of trustees. When he was asked about the lack of support of the faculty, and that before the offer to him was made final by the board, 2/3 of the faculty were against his candidacy. Since the board's decision at least 20 professors were still not in favor of the choice or the way it was handled. He reported that this was not his problem but between the board and the faculty.

Realizing that this line of discussion was getting nowhere we asked what his plans were. He replied that at the present he did not have an agenda but was asking questions of the RU faculty of where the University should go. We had a number of specific questions which I asked in a straightforward, calm and mature fashion. A brief synopsis is as follows:

We then asked if it was true that he was going to have a laboratory. His response was that he most definitely would. When asked about potential conflict of space, money or area he said that was ridiculous and that he believed that it would strengthen the University. G.B. asked whether this was wise since all presidents did not have laboratories because of the commitments of the presidency. He scoffed that our present president had many outside activities that he would not have.

When G.B. pressed this point by describing his own activities and how difficult it was to keep up, D.B. curtly responded that he was different and perfectly able to do all these things. He viewed the lab as his hobby. I then thought it appropriate to ask how much his commitment would be and how many outside activities he had. In the beginning he plans to spend 90% of his time here at the RU [breakdown between lab and presidency not discussed].

When asked about the question of the graduate program, he said that it would be impossible to have a university without it. It should be maintained. In fact, he thought it should be expanded. Perhaps more MDs should be encouraged to obtain a PhD.

D.B. was then asked about programs that he envisioned bringing in or strengthening. He replied with the following list in the order stated:

1. Yeast biology
2. Drosophilia biology
3. Mouse biology [When questioned he meant mouse genetics gene mapping and transgenic mice]
4. Neurobiology/behaviour
5. Structural biology

He then asked us what we wanted. We replied chemistry, immunology, biochemistry physicians for the hospital, biomedical scientists.

This part of the interview, of over an hour, was very constructive and informative.

At this point—asked if he would give us his views on the background to the Cell paper. D.B. responded in a rage and said that there was nothing seriously wrong with the paper and that who in fact said this. He then went from G.B. to A.C. to Z.C. demanding who on the faculty would read and understand this paper. After several moments of haranguing and confrontational posturing I pointed out to D.B. that his behaviour was exactly what we were worried about. He didn't understand this so I said that it was not easy to tell someone that they had bad breath but someone should tell him. It was pointed out for the previous hour we had had a constructive interaction that was carried out at an adult level. He was now behaving in an infantile fashion that wasn't appropriate or called for. We could have discussed this problem in the same adult fashion. He then apologized and said he would tell us whatever we wanted to hear or behave. I told him that it was not my job to follow him around to prompt him or what to say. He then calmed down and gave a brief but not very informative description of the case.

At the end of the meeting Z.C. thanked him for coming to visit with us and share his views. At which time he departed to a meeting with F.——

G.B., Z.C., and A.C. had further discussion after D.B. left. We all agreed that we had not been swayed from our opposition to D.B. candidacy to president. The following are problems that we noted.

1. D.B. openly displays hostile, angry and aggressive stances at inappropriate times. His arrogance definitely interferes.
2. The dual role of presidency and lab head is going to lead to conflict within the University and not going to allow time for the task of president. Being president needs a full time committed individual.
3. His fund raising ability is unknown and not obvious if he will be successful.
4. View of the future extremely narrow and not fitting for a university.
5. Ability to head the RU faculty is further doubted.

In 1990, The Rockefeller University was an institution in turmoil, and while almost everything that the new president proposed quickly became controversial in one way or another,[48] Cerami felt politically sidelined, that his views had been overlooked by David Rockefeller, and that ultimately his own power and influence was only going to diminish. Depressed at the thought of losing his autonomy and having to work within a dysfunctional scientific regime, Cerami sought solace in friends outside The Rockefeller University. One evening in 1990, while having dinner at Sandro's Restaurant on the Upper East Side with Richie Proper, a former business colleague, Jeffry Picower walked up to their table and was introduced to Cerami by Proper. Picower, a "publicity shy"[49] wealthy Florida-based philanthropist, wanted to expand his investment portfolio into the potentially lucrative biomedical research sector. Over the following months, Cerami and Picower devised a plan to establish a completely new biomedical research institute with an initial budget of $10 million, which would be guided by a signally benevolent aim—"to find cures for the maladies that afflict humankind."[50] For Cerami, destiny was not just a matter of chance but of choice, and he told a newspaper journalist that he "would have remained at The Rockefeller University if the opportunity to head a new institute had not come along."[51]

Picower appeared to be the source of the *geld* (money) that Ehrlich had prescribed as a necessary component for the successful pursuit of scientific work. Like Ehrlich, Cerami was a scientific gambler; then again, so too were a great many of the earlier microbe hunters, and he was also fired with a scientific intuition and single-mindedness to discover new pathogens. In the fall of 1990, Cerami began a new adventure by uprooting himself together with his entire team of thirty researchers and relocating to the newly instituted Picower Institute for Biomedical Research at North Shore University Hospital in Manhasset, Long Island. Cerami never thought that the day would come when he would leave The Rockefeller University, but as he stood on the corner of York Avenue and 62nd Street and looked back up the hill to the building in which Bronk had inspired his scientific heart three decades before, he felt anxious about the future. Should he have fought harder to stay? Was this an act of needless self-excommunication born of hubris? He wasn't to know that David Baltimore's ill-fated presidency was only to last a mere eighteen months and be regarded as the "stormiest 2 years in the Rockefeller's history."[52] Leaving was in truth a momentous move, but he had a profound belief in his own ability to re-create himself anew. He would try to build something that was the equal of The Rockefeller University with the gifted team of researchers that he had assembled. And in Jeffry Picower he believed that he had the support of a trusted patron working in tandem with a board of directors that contained some of the titans of twentieth-century U.S. business rectitude acting as guarantors of propriety, which included, among their number, Bernard L. Madoff. As he left The Rockefeller University for the last time after twenty-eight years, his sense of optimism was troubled; this was a critical time in his life, and he was haunted by the uncertainty that future gain would not compensate for this loss. Then, in one movement, he turned on his heels and walked away.[53]

10 · PHILANTHROPY GOES AWRY

> An active field of science is like an immense intellectual anthill; the individual
> almost vanished into the mass of minds tumbling over each other, carrying
> information from place to place, passing it around at the speed of light.
> —Lewis Thomas (*The Lives of a Cell: Notes of a Biology Watcher*)

The Picower Institute for Medical Research was established during a
portentous time in the development of a U.S. national science policy. The debate
examining the scientific basis for the support of biomedical science can be traced
to an article cowritten in 1976 by the cardiologist Julius Comroe and the anesthe-
tist Robert Dripps.[1] Their call for more research to be done on the nature of
research stemmed from a conspicuous asymmetry between the pace of basic science and the application of new knowledge to human problems.[2] The authors set
out to examine "whether the federal government would get more for its biomedical research dollars if they were used to support clinically orientated research or if
they were used to support research that was not clinically orientated." As an experiment, Comroe and Dripps scrutinized how the most important discoveries in
cardiovascular and pulmonary diseases were made. The equivocal finding of their
study was that 41 percent of over 500 key articles that led to advances were written
by scientists who had no interest in disease. But before thinking that this was a
ringing endorsement of research motivated solely by curiosity and without concern for application, they also found that more than half the papers were the result
of targeted clinical research.[3] Comroe and Dripps did not fully answer the conundrum, but the question facing the policy makers in Washington, D.C. was how best
to develop a proper applied science—and if this should be allowed to occur naturally, as a matter of course, or whether it can be ordered up more quickly, under
the influence of management and money. Comroe and Dripps ended their 1976
paper with a reasoned injunction: "We believe that a $2 billion industry [the
National Institutes of Health (NIH) budget was over $7 billion in 1990] might
well put more of its annual budget into research on improving its main product,
which in this case is discovery and its application."

Translating discoveries made in the lab to application in the clinic was the central purpose of the Picower Institute for Medical Research. When interviewed in
1991, Jeffry Picower outlined the guiding philosophy of the venture. "Basic science

doesn't necessarily have an application, ours starts with the application of a particular disease."[4] What defined Cerami was his curiosity and his imagination,[5] qualities he would use to apply modern scientific methods to medical problems. The new institute, under Cerami's scientific direction, was going to focus on finding therapies for the cure and prevention of a wide range of specific diseases, including malaria and other parasitic diseases, atherosclerosis and cardiovascular diseases, disorders of the central nervous system, tumors, cancers, and infectious diseases. The one insidious disease that preoccupied the minds of both Picower and Cerami was diabetes. When they were first introduced to each other in Sandro's restaurant, they had discovered that both of their mothers had died from complications arising from diabetes. Indeed, Jeffry Picower suffered from diabetes, as had his father before him. Thus, the work of Helen Vlassara's team, looking at the biochemical basis of the complications of aging and similar changes in diabetics, fitted perfectly into the prospective research corpus.

The relationship between scientists and capitalists, especially those with a hands-on approach to philanthropy, can be a complicated matrix for the scientist to navigate. Rarely is there a perfect synergy of motivation, purpose, utility, or validation. Cerami had been fortunate in being able to bring $2 million in NIH funding with him in existing grants to the new enterprise, and Picower's public statements seemed to indicate the moral righteousness of his own philanthropic vision. "When you're fortunate and you have the opportunity to give back to society," Picower told the *New York Times*, "and you meet someone like Tony, who's a world-class scientist, then from the ability that I have on the financial side and Tony's ability on the science side comes a natural partnership. . . . It's just for the benefit of science, and my family will not get anything back, no matter what happens."[6]

These were exciting days for Cerami, and relocating his entire team of highly prodigious medical "explorers" from The Rockefeller University to North Shore University Hospital was an opportunity of a lifetime. Intriguingly, he also viewed his strategically tailored multidisciplinary approach as something of a novel scientific experiment in itself. Experience had taught Cerami that laboratories often fail because their scientists never talk to each other, so his new project was conceived as one big "continual laboratory with no walls in between," where specialists would be interchangeable and the research approach interactive. These scientific ideals and crystalline research principles may have positioned the institute in the vanguard of translational medicine, but the early realities of daily life for the team in the two upper floors of the Boas-Marks Research Center were a world apart from the Tower Building overlooking the East River. But what blazes a trail is not necessarily pretty.

In 1991, when Cerami and his team arrived to occupy their 30,000 square feet of office space, they found it entirely empty, apart from their belief system. Cerami, over the previous decade, had encouraged his scientific staff to be courageous, honest, and dedicated to finding ways to help people who were sick. One of the methods he had used to fully immerse his staff in this belief and to create a sense of togetherness was the introduction of "beer and science Fridays" and, for the more discerning, "wine and science Fridays." These were "fantastic"[7] social gatherings held between 5 and 7 in the evening, where the cross-disciplinary team congregated to talk science, which helped to form the bonds of friendship. This feeling of pride and mutual loyalty shared by members of the group was to serve them well in the early days of the institution's life. In part, as a response to the trauma of leaving The Rockefeller University, there developed almost immediately a collective devotion to the Picower Institute. It rapidly became the center of their lives, cemented by gossip in bars and restaurants, making plans for the future, and building a determination to succeed. However, the first problem was getting from Manhattan, where most of the researchers lived, to Manhasset, on Long Island. Fortunately, Cornell University ran a shuttle bus service for its medical students to North Shore Hospital, which Cerami's staff could use. Two dynamic younger members of Cerami's scientific staff who made the morning journey from Manhattan were Annette Lee and Barbara Sherry. When both of the scientists arrived at 350 Community Drive, they would sit on the dusty floor of the nascent laboratory sorting applications into big piles as a first step in a recruitment process. Their task was to build a laboratory without walls that would place chemists next to biologists and scatter virologists among infectious disease specialists with the objective of increasing productivity and synchronizing research.[8] This construction of a distinct culture shaped the Picower Institute's scientific dynamic, which became based around a large collection of postdocs. Many were from the United States, but more than twenty came from Germany and others from Japan, Italy, and even one organic chemist from the West Bank, via Jordan and the University of Tubingen. Lee and Sherry were products of Cerami's scientific pedagogy and devoted to research paths that would provide targets for new diagnostics or new therapies. By the force of his personality, Cerami created an exciting scientific environment[9] and drove the translational process forward with a philosophical breadth and conceptual depth.

If Cerami was going to build a research institute that would satisfy his own ambitions and those of his scientific successors, then what was required was a program of bold adventures and initiatives to make it stand out from the crowd. As Barbara Sherry recalls, "Tony was not afraid to have an idea that seemed really crazy, if there was something new and outside the box, he wasn't afraid to pursue it. As a matter of fact, they were the only things he seemed interested in."[10] One of his seemingly outlandish ideas was to establish a new scientific journal that would have an emphasis on the importance of molecular medicine in understanding, diagnosing, treating, and preventing human diseases. This would be an undertaking of Harveian proportions. But who could Cerami entrust such an important task to? It would require someone with limitless creative energy, a person with a love and knowledge of literature and who possessed the editorial skills of a Robert B. Silvers. He did not have to look far. When Cerami became president of the Picower Institute for Medical Research (PIMR) in 1991, he soon hired his close friend and mentor Kenneth S. Warren. After Warren's expulsion from the Rockefeller Foundation, he had spent an eventful period as director of science at Maxwell Communications Corporation in New York City.[11] In 1992, with his enthusiasm for life still intact after the Maxwell hiatus, Warren joined the PIMR as vice president of academic affairs. As an original champion of biomedical sciences and an outlier for the concept of open access, he was ideally suited to his new role. In 1994, after two years of long and patient labor, Warren cofounded the journal *Molecular Medicine* and acted as its deputy editor.[12] For Cerami, the journal had a partly redemptive quality, acting as a remedy to the frustrations he felt while on the editorial board of The Rockefeller University's *Journal of Experimental Medicine* (*JEM*). In the 1980s, the *JEM* was justifiably recognized as the world's leading immunology journal, and when the formidable Henry Kunkel asked Cerami to join the editorial board to help expand *JEM*'s biomedical coverage, he accepted the challenge with alacrity. However, he did not feel that he had succeeded in moving *JEM*'s center of gravity toward molecular biology and therapeutic end points. Now, in a new institution and as editor-in-chief of the *Molecular Medicine* journal, he had a platform to showcase the new ideas and discoveries that would provide an educational foundation for the new generation of physician-scientists who he wanted to recruit into translational medicine.

Joined-up thinking was the scientific mantra of the PIMR, and rather than bemoan the loss of gifted medics to the discipline of translational medicine, Cerami accepted that it was up to scientists like himself to create the enthusiasm and the environment for productivity that is fun and satisfying above all. To that end, as an evocation of the MD-PhD program Cerami had established with Cornell University Medical School a decade before, he put all of his considerable efforts into establishing a PhD program for medical doctors at his new institution. The objective was to offer MD graduates a program that would encourage further laboratory studies in biochemistry and molecular biology and enable them to learn how to apply knowledge of basic science to medical problems at the bedside.

As a first step, the Education Department of the State of New York had to be persuaded that the new institution possessed the academic infrastructure to run such a novel program. Cerami had developed with his close colleagues a clear scientific understanding of the curriculum and concepts that would be required to offer a highly sophisticated teaching program at their new Graduate Medical School on Long Island. It was all to play for. On a snowy winter's morning in late December 1991, Cerami, together with Kirk Manogue and Annette Lee, drove over one hundred miles north, to Albany, the capital of New York, to present their new program to a specialist committee of the Education Department. Perhaps it was due to Cerami's focused determination and his firm conviction that a physician doing clinical work should also carry out their own laboratory investigations, but the charter was subsequently granted, and not only that, it was approved "into perpetuity"[13] by the Regents of the University of the State of New York to award a PhD in the field of molecular medicine. Both the journal of *Molecular Medicine*[14] and the Graduate School[15] are enduring achievements established in the early 1990s under Cerami's determined stewardship.

From the outset, the productivity and diversity of the research[16] at the Picower Institute were impressive and owed much to Cerami's continued ability to offer his protégés inspiration and protection from the harsh, buffeting realities of pursuing a scientific career suffused by the ethical values of free enterprise capitalism. The research program continued to be guided by Cerami's search for the chemical underpinnings of biological processes. This, after all, was what had led to his breakthrough in protein modification in HbA1c. A tangible outcome of Cerami's mentorship was the research program on macrophage migrating inhibitory factor (MIF), one of the first cytokine mediators to have been discovered, which among other things, is overexpressed in a number of cancer types.[17] For the rheumatologist Richard Bucala, the personal warmth and problem solving attitude in the lab were defining and led to "a special scientific environment created by Tony—it was exciting," and had the added benefit of fermenting an adhesive camaraderie within the group. Indeed, so formative was the experience on the career development of a cadre of young researchers that the chain of memory continues to be strengthened by regular meetings of what is known today as the International MIF Symposium. The first symposium was held at Trinity College Dublin in 2006 and reunited Bucala, Robert Mitchell, Seamas Donnelly, and Jurgen Bernhagen from Cerami's laboratory, with a new generation of researchers from across the globe for an extensive program of lectures on the biology and pathophysiology of MIF proteins and their receptors.[18] The influence of Cerami's scientific perspicacity continued to pulse outward, like a pebble in a pond, in ever increasing concentric circles.

In 1992, Cerami's contribution to discovery science and translational medicine was recognized by his election to the nation's preeminent scientific institution, the National Academy of Sciences. At the presentation ceremony, the president Frank Press read this citation: "Cerami's ability to integrate chemistry and biology lead to the recognition of the importance of the complexing of carbohydrates with protein in aging and to the discovery of the humoral mechanism by which tumors cause cachexia in the host."[19] Cerami's personality, imagination, and curiosity had made him into a scientific superstar. It appeared that he had the world at his feet. However, the world had other ideas.

Just like generations of scientists before him, Cerami thought that he too was realistic in his beliefs about how best to pursue biomedical research within a capitalist value system. And perhaps the emotional pain and distress of the departure from The Rockefeller University, together with the chance to relaunch his career in such a stellar fashion, clouded his judgment and made him less circumspect about the moral and financial motives of Jeffry Picower. But there had been an early warning sign. After just four months, his friend and the institute's first dean, Miki Rifkin, resigned to take up a permanent post at Mount Sinai, and her departure was the first fissure in the foundations of the new world that he was constructing. Rifkin was much admired for her administrative and scientific skills; in fact,

David Baltimore had wanted her to stay on as dean under his presidency. How-ever, he was only willing to offer a year-on-year contract, and because of Rifkin's family responsibilities, this arrangement was unacceptable, so instead she joined the Picower Institute as a tenured member of the academic community. But within a short time, Rifkin felt morally alienated. "I didn't like it. It was just not my kind of atmosphere. It was very commercially driven—that was the way it was set up. It was academic, but I wanted to be in a more academic institution and at that point I went to Mount Sinai."[20]

The relationship between Cerami and Picower was not limited to a business–biology alliance; they saw each other socially too. Both of them lived on Park Ave-nue, and Cerami often visited Barbara and Jeffry Picower in their sumptuous apartment near 66th Street. During their many discussions contemplating matters of life and death, as well as the role of nature and nurture in common diseases, Cerami was constantly surprised by one aspect of Jeffry Picower's gastronomic behavior—his insatiable appetite for White Castle burgers. It wasn't that Picower would have his chauffeur drive him the nine blocks to the 57th Street burger restaurant—although it did appear incongruous to see a limousine, engine idling at the curbside, while square burgers were flipped—what troubled Cerami was that Picower was a diabetic and the famous "slider" burgers were damaging his health. Cerami's warnings of the dangers of poor diabetic control were continuously ignored by Picower, and incrementally, this meaty metaphor took on a symbolic significance that led to a growing moral unease between the two men that fatally undermined their relationship.

Cerami's ethical uneasiness centered around the financial underpinnings of the Picower Institute and what he saw as a conflict of interest between Jeffry Picower's stated philanthropic principles and his for-profit business goals. Possibly naively, on one occasion, Cerami enquired of Picower exactly what amount of money he thought would be enough money for what he needed to do, and Picower replied, "I never have enough."[21] Cerami increasingly began to see a dark side of Jeffry Picower's allure and, from that moment on, saw him as a Midas figure dedicated to the endless accumulation of wealth. Certainly, in comparison to the philanthropic giants of Carnegie and Rockefeller, Picower appeared to be a one-dimensional, morally ambivalent, and lusterless humanitarian. It was Andrew Carnegie who stated that his aim was the "advancement and diffusion of knowledge and under-standing"[22] and originated the idea of the gift into perpetuity. Again, it was Carnegie who inspired the field of modern philanthropy by declaring that money amassed by modern capitalists was not ultimately for their personal purposes but rather that they held the funds in trust for the public and therefore should return those funds to the public. In his 1889 essay *Wealth*, Carnegie asserted that "the man who dies thus rich dies disgraced." In a similar vein, John D. Rockefeller's 1913 philan-thropic initiative was guided by the idea that money should be used for the benefit of humankind and that the best use of philanthropic giving should be measured by its ability to advance knowledge of the root causes of societal problems—for

Cerami, this was using biomedical science to ameliorate the human condition. However, it became increasingly apparent to Cerami that altruism had been subordinated to the profit motive in Jeffry Picower's distorted view of what constituted philanthropy.

The Picower Institute was established as a not-for-profit philanthropic entity founded on the concept that licensing and commercial income would accrue to support the discovery phase of the translational process. In that way, any profits would come back into the institute to support scientists in their search for new diagnostics and drug therapies. Alas, ethical standards had gone awry, and Cerami came to believe that his vision was being subverted by Picower, who had clandestinely spun out the intellectual property of the tax-exempt institute, secreting it away in his own for-profit companies. This left Cerami in an invidious position: knowing that the Picower Institute for Medical Research would end up with a reduced stake in any future profits from the pharmaceutical research they had helped to fund.[23] The perceptive Miki Rifkin's heightened suspicions had indeed been well grounded: Jeffry Picower's modus operandi was to commercialize philanthropy in order to make more money.

With little chance of scrutiny, Picower, who was portrayed in one newspaper as a "very sophisticated investor and hardball businessman,"[24] developed an ingenious business plan that interlinked his charitable organization and his for-profit goals. In 1993, Picower established his Pennsylvania-based Cytokine PharmaSciences, a for-profit pharmaceutical company. This company licensed many of the most promising patents developed by Picower's nonprofit medical research institute. Among the discoveries registered by the Picower Institute were patents for a molecule named CNI-1493, a drug that showed promise as an anti-inflammatory.[25] This complicated business strategy put Picower in a position to profit personally from drug research funded through his nonprofit institute. Little wonder, then, that Cerami came to regard Picower as a man of diaphanous morals and, in retrospect, with highly dubious business associates. The Jeffry M. and Barbara Picower Foundation was created in 1989 with its assets managed by Bernard Madoff from his offices on the 17th Floor of an office block, dubbed the "Lipstick Building" due to its design, in Midtown Manhattan. Madoff was the former investment adviser and orchestrator-in-chief of the largest Ponzi scheme in history and the most significant financial fraud in U.S. history at that time, estimated at over $64 billion.[26] Rather than being the savior of humanitarian ideals, it turned out that Jeffry Picower was an impenitent parvenu in the world of U.S. philanthropy, and his eponymous institute felt like a sinkhole opening under Cerami's feet. He felt betrayed.[27] Resources were supposed to be used for the benefit of society, and when he discovered the truth, he confronted Picower telling him, "You can't do this." After this tempestuous episode with Picower, Cerami was steadfast in his belief that biomedical science had a responsibility not only for the cure of the sick and for the prevention of disease but also for the advancement of knowledge on which both depend. Now, he saw the Picower financial empire for what it was, a toxic nexus of wealth, power, and deceit, and he was determined to extricate himself from its dense machinations at the earliest opportunity. But he postponed his departure because of the death of close friend and confidant Kenneth S. Warren in September 1996.

The hypothermic Warren, who once described Cerami as "my friend and alter ego,"[28] died of malignant melanoma on September 18, 1996, at his home in Dobbs Ferry. He was sixty-seven years old and had dedicated his life to improving the health of the world's poorest people. Warren's cancer had originally presented twenty years earlier, but conceivably as a result of diligently self-administering the BCG vaccine, he succeeded in gaining an extra twenty years of life. In celebration of Warren's enduring contribution to global health, Cerami organized an honorary degree ceremony for him at the Picower Institute on June 19, 1996. The occasion brought together a great vintage of friends and collaborators to celebrate Warren's life scientific and dedication to parasitology. This was an event of great lyricism for Cerami and acted as a counterbalance to what he saw as the nightmare of Picower's venality.

The breaking point for Cerami arrived on September 9, 1996, when he faxed a letter to Jeffry and Barbara Picower:

Dear Jeff and Barbara

After considerable thought and discussion I have decided to resign from being the President of The Picower Institute for Medical Research, as of September 15, 1996.

The stress of the past few years has taken a toll on my health that I do not wish to continue. . . .

I will, of course, continue my participation with Alteon on their research programs and related business activities. In addition, I may consult with other pharmaceutical and biotechnology companies in areas that I have expertise.

On September 25, in another fax, this time to the board members of the Picower Institute (which included Bernard L. Madoff), Cerami wrote, "After considerable thought and reflection, I have decided to resign from the Board of Trustees of The Picower Institute. The last thing that my successor needs is to have me on the Board second-guessing his or her decisions." On a somewhat curious note, he ended the letter with this sentence: "I know that you will continue to give excellent counsel to the Institute into the next millennium." This comment may well be explained by the imbalance of power and the calculus of damage limitation that Cerami felt for the friends and colleagues he was going to leave behind. Five years earlier, Cerami had arrived at Manhasset with his thirty-strong team of research workers, but he would be leaving entirely alone. Cerami's life was marked by periods of emotional and scientific oscillation, and his friend Charles Dinarello thinks that the Picower experiment led to his friend's partial withdrawal from the world. "I think Tony was not aggressive enough with Baltimore, and it was the beginning of a decline . . . and the Picower was going to be every bit as good as

The Rockefeller University, that was his intention. He had money, he had amassed all these wonderful people. . . . If I had to say what cataclysmic event made him withdraw it must have been the Picower, I think he got burned by that. He was betrayed."[29]

Motivation is one of the most important sentiments in science, and Cerami felt that his efforts to discover new ways to treat disease had been denigrated. Cerami referred to his five years as the president of the Picower Institute for Medical Research as "a very strange interlude in my life." He was no longer happy and not the kind of person to stay in a bad situation and waste time.[30] And in a stunning *coup de theatre*, he abruptly left the Picower Institute in an act of self-protection, bringing down the curtain on an experiment that barely five years before he thought would be his salvation. Seventy years earlier, when Martin Arrowsmith had been educated, painfully, in the ways of the world, he took himself off to the country-side to work in a homemade laboratory. In 1996, Cerami was equally attracted to this restorative path, and he too set off for the bucolic uplands to work in a home-made laboratory in pursuit of scientific truth and in accordance with his true self.

11 · TRANSLATION
IN TRANSITION

> Nature by herself determines all diseases and is herself sufficient in all things
> against all of them.
>
> —Thomas Sydenham, 1624–1689

The ability to theoretically understand a biological process before it is experientially established can be invaluable to the process of advancing scientific thinking. This capacity, together with what could be described as the usefulness of incomplete knowledge, had helped to establish Cerami as a leading translational scientist by the mid-1990s. Being constantly watchful for hypothetically plausible patterns was the method Cerami used to approach a scientific mystery. This was his obsession: to find the first elusive piece of a puzzle that might lead to a novel discovery, however undulating the path of chaotic coincidences or random the events may prove. Indeed, Cerami was not alone in deploying this methodological approach to finding scientific solutions, as the eminent American historian of science, Thomas S. Kuhn, noted just such a characteristic of the scientific temperament three decades before in his influential publication *The Structure of Scientific Revolutions*. "What then challenges him is the conviction that, if only he is skilful enough, he will succeed in solving a puzzle that no one before has solved or solved so well."[1]

Cerami still had an unshakable fidelity to his vocation—drug discovery—which he was determined to pursue. And in those early months of freedom from the emotional maelstroms of the Picower Institute for Medical Research, he felt "relieved beyond belief," even if leaving had produced painful shockwaves that destabilized—in some cases permanently—personal and professional relationships. Now, at least, the most hurtful and bitterly contested duplicities were gone—notably, the $100 million that Jeffry Picower promised[2] for medical research but that had never materialized. Picower's stance was so implacable that even Bernie Madoff's serial imploring, "Come on Jeff, put up more money,"[3] failed to persuade the parvenu patron to honor his pledges. Ultimately, the imbalance of power and the calculus of damage limitation forced Cerami to remove himself from what he increasingly recognized was becoming dangerous in his life.[4] Leaving was therefore an act of self-protection. In a dramatic way, he had brought a curtain down on a formative episode in his career, and it was to prove an Iron Curtain, an impenetrable divide, which encapsulated the trend of bridge burnings, schisms, and excommunications that came to define his personality and the trajectory of his life in science. At times, it was almost as if he did not possess a mechanism for bridging the gaps that connect the natural episodes of life. It was also widely recognized that Cerami was incapable of dedicating himself wholeheartedly to a project unless he was totally captivated—if a research question was not intellectually compelling, then he could not find solid ground in his world.[5] This feature of his character would lead him to break up relationships, veer off in unexpected directions, or team up with the wrong people.[6] In retrospect, one of Cerami's greatest scientific regrets was leaving the irreplaceable Kirk Manogue behind at the Picower Institute for Medical Research. Manogue was not only his trusted friend and "consigliere"[7] but also a discerning observer of the scientific landscape who possessed the vital nuanced skills necessary to orchestrate, manage, and maximize scientific creativity in the laboratory setting. In the years that followed, this absence was to have a powerful presence.

In 1996, what Cerami needed most was time to think. His life had oscillated between a desire to be surrounded by his fellow scientists in the noble pursuit of using science in the interests of humanity and wanting a life of isolation, free from disruptive institutional forces. Having seen how philanthropic ideals could atrophy or even vanish entirely, he now wanted to be liberated from exploitation and embrace the ethos of self-reliance and independence that Dr. Gottlieb had extolled to Martin Arrowsmith in the fictional McGurk Institute of Biology: "Work twice as hard as you can, and keep people from using you."[8]

Cerami's opportunity to begin a new life as an independent scientist came in the late summer of 1996 when his daughter, Carla, finished her MD/PhD training at NYU. Carla wanted to try something different from the conventional academic medicine career path, so they decided on a bold adventure, to set up their own not-for-profit research institute. In honor of Ken Warren, who had died on September 18, 1996, and in recognition of his scientific courage and daring, it was decided to call the new laboratory the Kenneth S. Warren Institute (KSWI). Money for translational research had always been hard to come by, and not even the exceptional long-term economic uptick during the years of the Clinton administration was sufficient to persuade investors to offer the funds required to undergird a well-planned program of biomedical research. This shortfall forced Cerami to take on consultancy work with a number of pharmaceutical companies that provided a lifeline during the financially precarious early period of the institute's existence. The initial failure to attract large grants from industry was hugely consequential and compelled Cerami to postpone his dream of locating the new laboratory in a rural idyll; instead, he and Carla established the KSWI in a former Union Carbide research complex in the town of Greenburg, Westchester County, New York.

Cerami's real skills were in getting things started, and historically, to push translational science forward, he needed a dedicated staff that he could lean on to help develop the new ideas that his insights and fits of mania would produce. Very soon, one of his trusted scientific collaborators, Peter Ulrich, joined the institute, and crucially, after giving a lecture at the Yale School of Medicine, Cerami met Mike Brines, a former Rockefeller graduate.[9] The meeting proved fateful and marked the beginning of a prodigious scientific collaboration. Brines, a tall, scholarly physician-scientist, was becoming disillusioned with his career as an endocrinologist at the Yale School of Medicine, and as he listened to Cerami's lecture, he became intrigued by the scientific potential of the KSWI. After the lecture, Cerami and Brines had an animated discussion about the role of translational science in modern medicine, and it was decided there and then that Brines should join the new enterprise. There was an instant chemistry between the two men, and a key factor to their relationship was that they had much in common. In addition to both being graduates of The Rockefeller University, they were punctilious, skilled experimentalists and had a shared biomedical vision: to try to understand what is wrong with people when they are sick and to develop cost-effective treatments.

To develop a free-standing laboratory requires capital, and this cannot always be met internally as the length of time between product conception and launch is both long and risky. The question facing every biomedical startup is simple and unequivocal—what are they going to be able to develop to sell? If the objective is a pharmaceutical, then a big investment in time and money is going to be required over a long period of time. The reality is that drug development is essentially the preserve of the pharmaceutical industry, because for a small-molecule drug or a biologic to be licensed by the Food and Drug Administration (FDA), it requires the scientific adjudication of highly expensive clinical trials to prove safety and efficacy if it is to be successfully translated from the laboratory to the clinic. An altogether less daunting pathway is to develop diagnostics. At this time, Cerami's dream, and business plan, was to discover another hemoglobin A1c–type assay that would be capable of providing the income stream and intellectual property rights to fund the acquisition of a research facility somewhere deep in the Westchester countryside. The idea of a laboratory in the woods, with its echoes of his life on the farm, had a deep emotional pull—there he imagined he would gain an understanding of the topography of his inner self and find the scientific knowledge that he could know nowhere else.

Remarkably, the early financial constraints, rather than inhibiting invention, brought the laboratory alive. As a follow-up to earlier work on advanced glycation end products (AGEs),[10] which suggested that tobacco smoke could generate cross-linking of proteins in the body and increase incidence of atherosclerosis and cancer in smokers, the research team hypothesized a method that would remove some of the harmful aqueous extracts in tobacco smoke.[11] Moreover, Cerami and his daughter established an ancillary company, Farrington Pharmaceuticals, to continue the work on the "breaker technology" products that were pharmacologically similar to aminoguanidine and other potential inhibitors of AGE formation. The company held patents on a range of inventions that proliferated throughout the late 1990s, including one for a controlled drug delivery device, and more infelicitous, for a filter that was designed to remove the reactive sugars and other harmful compounds from tobacco to offer a less poisonous cigarette.

On the eve of the millennium, Cerami's new laboratory included both a company and a basic research component and had succeeded in attracting a small and growing team of skilled experimentalists eager to contribute to projects in discovery science. The philosophy underpinning the lab's work was to investigate what Cerami categorized as three fundamental aspects of human disease: understanding, treatment, and prevention. Importantly, evidence amassed over his lifetime had taught him that most scientific breakthroughs arrived in unexpected ways and that to really discover things, imagination and criticism were fundamental components of scientific inquiry. Creativity also occupied a central position in his thinking, and it was Cerami's continued ability to see biological connections that others could not[12] that would open up new territory and bring about the conceptual breakthrough that moves our knowledge of human biology forward.

In marked contrast to the institute's accelerating scientific proficiency, the entire enterprise was frequently in danger of collapse due to hemorrhaging money it did not have. The desperate financial situation was in part compensated for by the team's spiritual adhesion to each other coupled to the excitement of working at the frontiers of discovery science. There was also a collective awareness that as a group, they were lucky to have so much intellectual freedom at a time when there was a conspicuous dwindling of outlets for individual initiatives and personal creativeness in the modern world of laboratory science. Mike Brines, who had rapidly taken on the mantle of the institute's brain trust, became increasingly aware of the potent contradiction that at once enriched and threatened the institute's existence. He found the day-to-day science exciting and fulfilling, but the institute was financially embattled with cash reserves at such dangerously low levels "that at times we were working on fumes."[13] Then, unexpectedly, economic salvation came in the form of a generous contract from Ortho Biotech, a subsidiary of the pharmaceutical behemoth Johnson & Johnson (J&J). Ortho Biotech wanted the KSWI to systematically examine the biological effects of their product erythropoietin (EPO),[14] the hormone that mediates red blood cell production, that had been developed as a treatment for anemia in patients with cancer. Thirty years previously, Cerami's first research project as an assistant professor in his own laboratory was to attempt to purify and determine the structure of erythropoietin from the urine of anemia patients. In 1969, EPO had not been isolated or characterized, and Cerami was determined that he would be the first person to do so. Alas, after two years of interminable failure and realizing that the project was in danger of ending his career before it had really begun, he admitted defeat and gave up the venture. Depressed and downcast,[15] it would be understandable if the EPO debacle had been willfully dispatched to the furthermost recesses of his memory. But now redemption beckoned—could EPO form another decisive moment in his life scientific? Cerami even wondered if perhaps the return to erythropoietin into his laboratory was somehow preordained. On the eve of his sixtieth birthday, he felt the forces of the past pressing him forward with surging velocity. He had been unable to solve the EPO puzzle three decades before, and now the mysteries of the protein hormone were to be confronted once again—*EPO Redux*.

Ortho Biotech (formally Ortho Pharmaceutical Corporation), a J&J wholly owned company, had been marketing and developing recombinant human erythropoietin (rhEPO)[16] in the 1990s and had grown the product from a sleepy, "several million-dollar pharmaceutical" into a $6 billion best-selling bioengineered drug.[17] Originally, rhEPO was developed for patients with renal insufficiency and renal failure, and it was later used to treat patients with anemia caused by cancer treatment.[18] At the time, the head of clinical and regulatory affairs at Ortho Biotech was oncologist Loretta Itri. Itri's profound interest in EPO was not simply professional; it was also deeply personal. In the late 1980s, Itri's mother died of pancreatic cancer, and during the final months of the illness, while nursing her mother, Itri became aware of a striking and pronounced feature of the disease: the total physical exhaustion and malaise that it caused. Gone from her mother was the seemingly unconquerable life-affirming maternal energy only to be replaced by listlessness and fatigue. The lethargy that resulted from her mother's illness informed Loretta Itri's scientific thinking and gave her valuable insights into deciphering disease processes. In the early 1990s, the accepted biomedical rationale was that the administration of rhEPO encouraged a biological chain reaction that stimulated red blood cell production, which increased hemoglobin levels that, in turn, oxygenated cells and improved energy levels. However, this dose-response interaction began to be questioned at the end of the decade, when Itri, as part of her program of monitoring the effectiveness of EPO, talked to a cohort of nurses who routinely treated patients with cancer. "The interesting observation that so many nurses began to report," Itri reflected, "was that patients who were receiving EPO seemed to feel better and get their energy back *before* their hemoglobin levels went up."[19] Thus, it appeared to Dr. Itri that EPO was producing other biological effects in addition to the production of red blood cells and to find out what these activities were would require an expert well versed in the causes of cachexia and anemia, a modern well-equipped laboratory, and a team of highly skilled experimenters.

It was no surprise that Itri would turn to Cerami to explore the EPO mystery, because he had been her scientific mentor since the 1970s, when she first worked in his laboratory during summer vacations while still a premed student at Long Island University. In the years that followed, Itri saw how Cerami worked tirelessly to gain an understanding of the pathology of human diseases and develop clinical strategies to conquer specific illnesses. "When he was developing TNF, he would frequently ask me," Itri explained, "what were the really big problems that I was seeing in the emergency room?"[20] Although Cerami was not medically qualified, his focus was on mechanisms of disease, and unlike physicians, who are, in the main, compelled to give answers and advocate a practical course of action at the bedside, Cerami could wait until he understood the natural history of a specific disease before advocating a strategy. Fundamentally, he wanted to know *why* diseases occurred and what could be done to prevent or cure them. By doing this, Cerami taught people how science could become an important force for social change. Exposure to this focused approach at the beginning of Itri's career in oncology transformed how she thought about the origins of disease, the immune system's response to infection, and the role of scientific discovery in medicine. During the intervening decades, Itri had ascended the medical-pharmaceutical hierarchy, gaining a level of financial autonomy that allowed her to commission long-term research projects that were clinically important. Of course, it also presented Cerami with an enticing biomedical puzzle, and he seldom walked away from a challenge. In fact, on the eve of the project, Loretta Itri felt fully vindicated in her choice of Cerami as the principal invesigator in the EPO study when she recalled a conversation that had taken place between them in the basement laboratory of Theobald Smith Hall twenty years before: "Tony has a unique way of looking at the world, a way of engaging directly upon the study of medical problems, which he described as: 'I have a constellation of known facts in front of me and it is when I have a piece of information that somehow doesn't fit, that's how I know where there is something I need to examine.'"[21]

When Cerami was given a grant to determine whether EPO directly affects cognitive function and well-being, the piece of information that intrigued him the most were the reports that patients "frequently perked up cognitively"[22] in advance of any increase in red blood cell numbers. This observation framed the design of a series of experiments based on the hypothesis that EPO might be interfering with TNF, which Cerami and his team knew could induce malaise in animals and people.[23] "We speculated," Mike Brines later wrote, "that EPO administered to these patients might reduce TNF-a production and hence improve cognition. Alternatively, EPO could directly affect cognition."[24] The task was to determine whether EPO, a large protein that, according to the prevailing scientific orthodoxy, could not cross the blood-brain barrier, had direct effects on the central nervous system. Previous experiments had shown that the peritoneal (abdominal) administration of TNF to rats caused the animals to take longer to learn a Morris water navigation maze. To the team's amazement, the animals given EPO learned the maze faster than animals given saline. From past experiments, Cerami knew that TNF played a role in promoting the damage of tissues due to stroke, head trauma, and eye and kidney damage. As a consequence, it was decided to see if EPO given intravenously could reduce the amount of damage in these tissues. After a year of experiments, the team reported[25] that EPO possessed biological activities in addition to the erythropoietic effects that originally provided its name. Moreover, they were able to show that peripherally injected r-Hu-EPO (recombinant human erythropoietin) could protect brain tissue from a variety of invasive procedures, including ischemia/hypoxia, as well as trauma. Thus, the work refuted the belief that the blood-brain barrier effectively excludes large glycosylated molecules such as EPO. Although exogenous EPO was effective, the puzzle for Cerami's team to solve was, what was its source in a living organism (in vivo)?

We have already seen how parallel discoveries happen in science, and while Cerami's group was the "advanced guard"[26] of the study of the nonerythropoietic effects of EPO, it was another group led by Satohiro Masuda[27] that provided the answer by demonstrating that glial cells derived from the nervous system produce EPO in response to hypoxia (a condition when the body is deprived of an adequate oxygen supply). This observation that EPO was made in the tissue surrounding the injury site constituted a "paradigm shift"[28] for the team, especially for Cerami, as he began to make biological sense of the evidence being amassed. His belief was that TNF evolved primarily as nature's antibiotic against invading bacteria and parasites. In this context, TNF generation by tissue surrounding the pathogen acts to sterilize the surrounding environment by initiating what Cerami terms "all-out war"[29] to destroy the invader. Since discovering cachectin/TNF in the 1980s, Cerami had been obsessed with trying to find the "shut-off valve" to the potent cytokine's destructive force, because seeing nature as an intrinsically balanced system, he was convinced that a biological antidote had symbiotically evolved. Cerami had proved that TNF contributed to inflammation, and as well as activatory receptors, he theorized that some brake on the system, in the form of inhibitory receptors, would also exist.[30] Otherwise, even small injuries like a bump on the head, or a small cut to a finger, could lead to devastating damage or death. For more than a decade, Cerami had searched for other cytokines made by macrophages that had either proinflammatory or anti-inflammatory action. During this period, his team identified a number of new proinflammatory cytokines but completely failed to discover any new anti-inflammatory molecules.[31]

Now, a sense of sudden enlightenment pulsed through Cerami's mind as he realized that EPO had the opposite biological profile to that of TNF; it decreased apoptosis and inflammation while improving the rate of healing and regeneration of tissue after damage. TNF and EPO appeared to be two sides of the same coin. In a connecting sequence of experiments, his team was able to show that EPO and TNF could regulate the production and activity of the other. Another revealing discovery, and one that explained why Cerami's previous attempts to find the mechanism that countered TNF-associated damage proved bathetic, was that he had been looking in the wrong place. He had assumed that the inhibitor would be produced by macrophages—it never occurred to him that surrounding cells would be the source and that the signal for local production of EPO is the activation of HIF-1[32] (hypoxia-inducible factors) by hypoxia that is caused by TNF impairing blood flow, as well as directly by inflammatory pathways.[33]

Theodosius Dobzhansky's aphorism that "nothing in biology makes sense except in the light of evolution"[34] had guided Cerami's team to a dramatic discovery— the method by which the body repairs itself. Feelings of excitement flowed through the corridors of the laboratory's animal facility and, working alongside the team,

Loretta Itri remembered it as "the best of times, and it was energizing because we knew that we were onto something incredibly important."[35] Energizing it certainly was, but the research was also viewed as being controversial on two separate counts. First, there was a strong opinion in the hematology world that EPO is a hormone that only does one thing—stimulates the production of red blood cells. Second, there was a mounting tension between Johnson & Johnson's R&D department and Ortho Biotech because the parent company felt that the type of discovery science being funded at the Kenneth S. Warren laboratory encroached upon their raison d'être. For his part, Cerami had grown used to the constant external pressures exerted on the discovery scientist: the struggle between money and science, between position and opposition, all intermingled with the internal, complex forces of his own personality: unbridled curiosity, ego, brilliance, narcissism, and a trenchant fear of boredom. Above all, excitement was to be harnessed, the new embraced, and the direction of travel was always into the future. Encouraged by solving the puzzle of EPO, and with seemingly endless and generous quarterly checks from Ortho Biotech, Cerami decided that it was time to relocate the Kenneth S. Warren Institute to a more fitting setting, one that would fulfill his ambition to explore biomedical science in a bucolic setting.

Just such an opportunity arose in the early spring of 2001, when Cerami and his daughter Carla bought a former research facility of the Brooklyn Botanic Gardens and fifteen acres of land from the Kitchanwan Institute near the town of Ossining, on the Hudson River. The resplendent early twentieth-century two-story building was over 16,000 square feet in size, allowing space for a laboratory, offices, and a small animal facility. The Kenneth S. Warren Institute's new home was set in a 180-acre wooded park owned by the county of Westchester, bordered by one of New York City's reservoirs. The scene was a magnificent evocation of Henry David Thoreau's rural idyll in his book *Walden; or, Life in the Woods*. The inviting quietness of Cerami's light-dappled office located deep in the woods should have prophesied a period of tranquility and meditative inner peace, but this was not a time of contentment; rather, it was a period of dark melancholy arising from the consequences of life and its desperations.

Helen Vlassara, Tony Cerami's second wife, did not follow him from the Picower Institute to the KSWI. They had been "mostly"[36] happily married for over twenty years, and scientific collaborators for even longer, until the gravitational force that had kept them together began to weaken. Over time, it seemed that Helen and Cerami's relationship had metamorphosed from being a loving couple into something more closely resembling scientific competitors. A bulletproof self-belief, the need to always be in charge, and an unwavering trust in one's own ideas are characteristics that can serve an investigator well in discovery science, but equally, they may jeopardize the flowering of the emotional intelligence and empathy necessary to sustain intimate relationships. After two decades, Cerami's marriage to Helen Vlassara ended in a bitter, exhausting, and protracted four-year divorce.[37] Ever more, Cerami became conscious of a great divergence in his life: he began to feel emotionally stagnant, lonely, and engulfed by threnodies of desolation and loss. He was becoming more detached—and dangerously unmoored. It was the Canadian psychoanalyst Elliott Jaques who was the first to use the term *midlife crisis* in 1965, and sure enough, Cerami's behavior began to change noticeably.[38] He seemed to have developed an aberrant hunger to be comforted and increasingly searched for solace in a series of relationships with much younger women. But rather than bringing the levity that he so craved, these short-lived romantic affairs brought the added complications of disillusionment and depression. Even some of his most stalwart supporters were worried that he was having a type of life crisis or emotional breakdown resulting from the removal of the social and professional mores to which he had grown accustomed.[39] Frequently, people are at their happiest when they are not thinking about themselves, when they are absolved of the need for self-analysis; alas, Cerami's psychological state during this period did not afford him this freedom. He felt confused and discombobulated as he searched to discover if the way he was living was timorous or bold.

This question was soon indisputably answered when Cerami met Colleen, a twenty-eight-year-old administrator, at a foundation board meeting. After a few months, on an impulse of affection, the couple married. Within a short time, in 2002, their daughter, Angelina, was born. Cerami, who was sixty-two years old, was overjoyed with the birth of his daughter, but unfortunately, the prediction made by many of his friends that the marriage would be short-lived proved correct. "From the get-go," Mike Brines saw the love affair as a disaster and one that caused Cerami "untold misery."[40] The couple were very poorly suited,[41] and as well as being emotionally draining, the evanescent relationship was to prove financially punitive for Tony Cerami. A prenuptial agreement had been signed by the couple, but it was poorly drafted, which led to lengthy, unpleasant, and expensive legal arbitration in front of a retired judge.[42]

Cerami loved and was equally devoted to all of his children, and at the KSWI, he now had the pleasure of working in a professional capacity with his physician-scientist daughter, Carla. Ethan and Carla were often seen running around the lab in The Rockefeller University,[43] and exposure to the concentrated intensity of scientific research played a part in directing Carla to medical school, to a dedication to parasitology and becoming a translational scientist in her own right. This scientific-familial dynamic was altered when Carla married Learned Jeremiah Hand, a self-proclaimed business guru and entrepreneur. Hand is a nephew of Judge Learned Hand, the reforming federal court judge, much admired for his tolerance and reputation as a defender of free speech and civil liberties during a divisive time in the history of the United States. In January 2000, Learned Jeremiah Hand joined the Cerami family business as vice president and chief operating officer for the KSWI, portraying himself as a modernizer with the necessary business acumen to expand the institute in new and ambition directions. Soon he spearheaded a major project for the KSWI with the launch of a new brand of cigarettes paradoxically named "Wellstone Filters," and the brand's unique selling point was the Cerami (and

Brines) designed filter that claimed to remove damaging toxins and carcinogens in tobacco. "People will buy it for the price," Jeremiah Hand confidently predicted, "and come back for the taste."[44] During the early years of Hand's involvement with the business–biology strategy of the KSWI, it became apparent that he was a hugely contradictory figure; while charismatic, outgoing, "suave,"[45] and a smooth operator, he was also unscrupulous, and his renunciation of the federal laws that oversee the ethical values of U.S. business practice would later bring about his downfall.[46] Learned Jeremiah Hand's confidence that Wellstone Filters could penetrate the highly lucrative U.S. cigarette market was short-lived, and when the product failed, leaving investors angry and out of pocket, his business ethics and role in the company came to be questioned. Distrust then turned to exasperation when Hand disappeared and was incommunicado for a week—he was rumored to be in Cuba—deserting his role as vice president, and when he finally returned, Tony Cerami had him unceremoniously fired. Understandably, the sacking of her husband "really really bothered Carla,"[47] and the event was so profoundly traumatic that it caused a painful estrangement between father and daughter that has not yet been reconciled. Up to that point, schisms, bridge burnings, and relationship breakdowns had been a powerful influence that forged and redirected the course of Cerami's life, sometimes for the better and sometimes not. The tragedy that unfolded was in part emotional, breaking as it did a bond between father and daughter, and scientific too, because the potential and excitement that ushered in their new endeavor was now diluted as Cerami and Carla went their different ways. Cerami had certainly been correct in seeing his son-in-law as a rapacious individual; once feted as a charismatic, genius dealmaker, Hand's fall was precipitous and ignominious. Capitalism and science are both human constructs, and Cerami had learned over the course of his career that they were best pursued with a tempering of realism. "When you work on the fringe," Cerami acknowledges, "you sometimes attract fringe people."[48]

Of course, just when it seems that things cannot get worse, they do. A large clinical study of recombinant erythropoietin (rhEPO) revealed that trauma patients admitted to intensive care units had a lower death rate but a significant increase in thrombotic (the forming of blood clots) events.[49] It appeared that the amounts of EPO that were required for tissue protection could also induce a procoagulation state that led to thrombosis.[50] Additionally, a concern was also raised that rhEPO could support tumor growth, the hypothesis being that by raising hemoglobin to a normal level, cancer cells might be able to create a self-sustaining blood supply. Conterminously, an alarming increase in the incidence of thrombosis was being seen in professional racing bicycle riders who used EPO to stimulate the production of erythrocytes to improve their performance. This escalating level of unease led to the US Food and Drug Administration adding a black box warning to the safety labeling for erythropoiesis-stimulating agents advising of the increased risk of death associated with their use in patients with cancer and renal failure. The FDA decision, while corporately damaging to Amgen and Johnson & Johnson, did not prove ruinous: as biotechnology giants, they had already made millions of dollars[51] from manmade versions of erythropoietin and possessed a broad, evolving portfolio of drugs and hi-tech medicines. Cerami and his team, however, did not have a fallback position; they had spent too much time and money to give up on the molecule. If EPO could not be used as a tissue-protective molecule in clinical medicine, they decided that their only way forward was "to go back to square one, and tear the molecule apart"[52] and see if it was possible to engineer a smaller EPO molecule so that it would not induce coagulation but still retained the tissue-protective activity.

In a series of painstaking experiments over a number of years,[53] the research group showed that rhEPO interacted with two receptors: the homodimer receptor, involved in the making of red blood cells and platelets, which was causing the coagulation problems, and the heteromer receptor of the erythropoietin receptor (EPOR) disulfide linked to the beta-common receptor CD131, which they named the *innate repair receptor*. It was found that this tissue-protective factor is generally not expressed by normal tissues but is upregulated immediately after injury. Once they knew that there were two receptors, then the question became whether they could find a ligand (a binding molecule) that would only bind to one and not the other. Subsequently, the team studied two EPO derivatives that were previously reported not to be erythropoietic in vivo. They discovered that Asialo-EPO can induce erythropoiesis in vitro but is completely inactive in vivo because of its extremely short half-life.[54] The biologist Sydney Brenner wrote, "I've always found it interesting to bring projects to the stage that other people can take them over and develop all the tricks,"[55] and one of Cerami's widely acknowledged "tricks" was carbamylation. And it was found that carbamylated erythropoietin (CEPO, which is made by the reaction of cyanate with the amino groups of EPO) is not erythoropoietic in vivo or in vitro. Employing the CEPO column, Cerami was able to isolate the tissue-protective receptor[56] to great effect.

One of the dedicated scientists working on the CEPO project was Thomas Coleman,[57] who joined the Kenneth S. Warren Institute in 2001, and straightaway became involved in one of the most exciting experiments of his entire career. "I was involved in the spinal injuries experiments, and when we put the animals on a treadmill, within two weeks, the CEPO dosed injured rats were indistinguishable from the uninjured animals. It was phenomenal."[58] This was the decisive proof that Cerami had been looking for, that CEPO, a nonerythropoietic, tissue-protective molecule, could offer significant advantages for the treatment of injury and disease. Equally, this was not a quixotic judgment; it was accepted that for the hypothesis to be successfully translated from the laboratory to use at the bedside, it "will require evaluation within the setting of clinical trials."[59] Inexorably, the research was moving into the R&D territory occupied by Big Pharma, as conducting expensive randomized controlled trials and making recombinant molecules were capital intensive ventures far beyond the resources of the Kenneth S. Warren Institute. In truth, it was astonishing how far they had come, but it was becoming vital, if they were to survive in the Darwinian world of translational science, that they commercialized their discoveries. At this point, they entered intensive discussions with J&J to establish a licensing agreement, with Loretta Itri acting as their emissary. "I tried to get the J&J management to license the small molecules that Tony had developed. But they were not interested. Misguidedly not interested."[60]

The rejection was a painful reminder of the realpolitik associated with pursuing translational science in the era of Big Pharma, and it came as a financial hammer blow leading to a cycle of declining remuneration at the KSWI, descending to half salary, then no salary, and the partial breakup of the research team. But what an impressive research team they had been! One of Cerami's major strengths was identifying good people and fitting them into a model that could function creatively at the frontiers of biomedical science. In addition, the disparate group eschewed the frills, status symbols, and unnecessary artifacts of discovery science. There was no insatiable appetite for ergonomically designed buildings, or futuristic apparatus, and no Rockefeller-type library—everything was done on the Internet. The whole enterprise was made up of little more than a dozen people: four PhD students, a couple of technicians, some administrative staff, and a critical mass of experimentalists. This core team was periodically augmented by collaborative partners from all over the world. One of the most unusual and industrious partnerships was with a gifted group of Turkish surgeons who worked continuously, in shifts, for a period of six months in the laboratory's animal facility. The arrangement was mutually advantageous, as the surgeons needed PNAS (Proceedings of the National Academy of Sciences of the United States of America) papers to get promotions in their home country but where they had no access to laboratory animals, and in return, the KSWI performed experiments around-the-clock, accumulating data that were needed to move research programs forward.[61]

Cerami had felt humiliated after the J&J debacle and redoubled his efforts to find a partner-investor with deep pockets. This quest, however, necessitated both a scientific and a business change of direction. Scientifically, Brines and Cerami had shown that the EPO involved in neuroprotection was not the same as the EPO used by the body to maintain red blood cell mass and therefore was different from the commercial EPO product.[62] This key realization indicated to the researchers that the tissue-protective effects of EPO were likely mediated by a different receptor than the one used by red blood cells.[63] The existence of this alternative receptor opened up the possibility that modification to the EPO molecule or synthesis of similar molecules might result in a molecule that interacted only with a tissue-protective receptor (which they later named the innate repair receptor [IRR]). This discovery led to a change in the business model being pursued; in order to commercialize inventions being made at the institute, Warren Pharmaceuticals, a for-profit entity, was formed in May 2001. In the same year, Cerami succeeded in forming a partnership with Lundbeck, a Danish pharmaceutical company. A Danish investment firm BankInvest and Warren Pharma licensed the cytokines to Lundbeck in the field of central and peripheral nervous system disorders. However, Cerami and Lundbeck entered the collaboration under a misapprehension—both failed to appreciate how difficult it was to make recombinant proteins. Lundbeck, for their part, had been a small-molecule company with little experience of the complex techniques required to produce "biologics." Lundbeck's business plan was to make its own version of EPO, thereby avoiding any patent infringement. Unfortunately, the clone that they used for EPO was not correct, making their end product unusable. At which point, Lundbeck senior management decided to cut their losses and terminate the agreement with Cerami, initiating yet another funding crisis for the KSWI group.

Financial catastrophe was only averted when Cerami and Mike Brines were able to enter into an agreement with Shire in October 2006,[64] a new biotechnology company formed in the United Kingdom in 1986 that focused on rare diseases and other highly specialized conditions. "Shire," as Mike Brines recounts, was an advanced biotech firm "who were making human EPO, almost in a generic way, and in a different method to that used by AMGEN and ROCHE. . . . Then there were legal issues, and in the end, Shire decided to get out of the EPO business and terminated their agreement with us."[65]

During this period of tumult, the development of tissue-protective proteins continued, which revealed that peptide fragments of EPO also activated the IRR. The agreement with Lundbeck allowed Warren Pharma to develop peptides smaller than 30 amino acids, and to do this, Warren Pharma spun out another entity, Araim Pharmaceuticals, in 2006. In a similar arrangement to that between KSWI and Warren Pharma, there was an understanding that Brines and Cerami would divide their time between the two commercial entities to ensure the goals of both corporations were coequal.[66] By this time, Cerami and his team had been experimenting with parts of the EPO molecule and found that asialo-EPO, which has an extremely short half-life in living organisms, had all the tissue-protective activity of EPO. This realization, as Cerami later wrote, "encouraged us to evaluate peptides as tissue-protective molecules."[67] Once again, Cerami found himself on the frontiers of the business–biology dynamic, and as he had learned from his experiences with TNF, there is a long timeline between the basic discovery being made and clinical studies being undertaken to determine whether the approach would be effective. To successfully translate novel peptides into approved drugs for clinical use would require considerable patience, time, and money. In 2006, Cerami was running out of all three.

12 · ANTI-TNF THERAPY
Changing the Pharmaceutical Landscape

Isolationism is over; we all depend upon and sustain each other.
—Peter Medawar (in A. Silverstein, *A History of Immunology*)

The failure of the biotechnology company Centocor to have its drug Centoxin approved by the Food and Drug Administration (FDA) for the treatment of Gram-negative sepsis not only brought the firm to the edge of bankruptcy[1] but also effectively ended Cerami's direct attempts to use monoclonal antibodies to block the activity of soluble ligands in the blood.[2] After making his indelible contribution to the science that underpinned anti-TNF therapy, Cerami, for a combination of reasons including arrogance, boredom, disappointment, and the enticing excitement of new scientific ventures, abdicated his lead position in the field. Radical as this may have been on a personal level, this was far from being seen as an act of scientific apostasy; other researchers who recognized the therapeutic possibilities that Cerami's research signified galvanized a massive effort to further investigate the potential of antibodies to block the activity of a secreted molecule in the blood.[3] Despite leaving the project to which he had dedicated so much time in search of new horizons, Cerami remains an integral part of the wider TNF story, not least because—as has been outlined previously—he was crucial in establishing the foundations upon which later research would be built. Exploring the later history and evolution of anti-TNF treatments underscores the real significance of this early work in setting up a field that has come to generate big pharma over $300 billion during the past twenty years and brought immeasurable improvements to the lives of the majority of people suffering from autoimmune diseases.

The discovery of anti-TNF therapy is a remarkable story of cutting-edge technological ingenuity that was needed to answer the problem that the pharmaceutical industry, with its focus on chemical drugs, had been unable to solve. Advances made in protein and genetic engineering, basic science, translational medicine, and the vital element of luck all coalesced to bring about a therapeutic revolution by establishing a new medical armamentarium—the biologics industry. The potent historical force of these components, while indispensable, does not, however, fully explain the success of anti-TNF therapy. Indeed, of equal importance was the human dimension: the competitive rivalries, combustible rejoinders, close friendships, and bonds of human chemistry formed over years of hard labor at the laboratory bench. These relationships and partnerships proved necessary to the timing and success of a treatment that "produced rich dividends in the form of therapies for chronic disease inflammatory diseases"[4] and transformed the lives of patients across the world.

One of the elements that transcended the sepsis failure in 1991, and the spectacular success in the late 1990s of anti-TNF therapies in the treatment of many chronic inflammatory disorders, including Crohn's disease, severe plaque psoriasis, and rheumatoid arthritis, was the anti-TNF antibody cA2 developed in the laboratory of Jan Vilcek. After defecting from Czechoslovakia in 1964, Vilcek, who trained as a virologist, joined the faculty of New York University Medical School and remained there for his entire career. In 2014, I visited Vilcek in his office high above the East River, and as the ferries crisscrossed the waterway between Manhattan and Queens far below us, Vilcek described the undulating path of scientific discovery and how his lab developed the first TNF inhibitor approved for clinical use. "Cerami and Beutler had showed that TNF is a key factor in the development of sepsis, and we made a monoclonal antibody in anticipation that it might be helpful in sepsis in collaboration with Centocor."[5] The ability to overcome technological hurdles was a crucial factor in the evolution of anti-TNF therapeutics, and a central figure in that collective effort was Junming "Jimmy" Le, a talented postdoctoral researcher working in Vilcek's laboratory. Le had grown up in China during the tumultuous years of Mao Zedong's Cultural Revolution, and after a period at Sloan Kettering Cancer Center, New York, where he was involved in making monoclonal antibodies, he joined Vilcek's team in the early 1980s. "Jimmy was very productive," remembered Vilcek, "and he was actually the person who produced the original mouse monoclonal antibody to TNF in our laboratory."[6] The cA2 TNF inhibitor was then passed to Centocor—who had paid for the research work—and under the supervision of J. N. "Jim" Woody, the company's chief scientific officer, the mouse antibody was chemerized[7] to reduce immunogenicity in humans as part of the preparation for the clinical trial in sepsis, inspired by Cerami and Beutler's earlier observations.

Although the agent was an extremely powerful TNF-a blocker, the clinical trials carried out in 1991 failed the test of efficacy, as there was no statistically significant improvement in patients during the course of the disease. More positively, there were no adverse side effects reported, and the antibody was well tolerated. But as a potentially effective therapeutic, it appeared as if cA2 had died a natural death: "At that point," reflected Vilcek, "we all felt that this was the end of the road, and we didn't have any bright ideas."[8] Understandably, this failure of the chimeric antibody to be approved for clinical use in the treatment of sepsis elicited consternation among the burghers of the balance sheet on Wall Street who had bet heavily on the success of the biologic drug. The economic ramifications were immediately felt at Centocor's headquarters in Malvern, Pennsylvania, and the company's stock price nosedived precipitously, falling from $60 to $6 in a day,[9] forcing the company to lay off staff, including a salesforce that had been hired in anticipation of the drug's success.[10]

Fortunately, Centocor's corporate retrenchment left Jim Woody's scientific team and his promising research program relatively unaffected. As has been recorded, translational medicine can, on occasion, be a hothouse of feuds, intrigues, and jealousies; likewise, it can be the canvass upon which close personal and professional friendships thrive. Indeed, it was this nexus of friendship that had been built up over many years, together with the feeling of being part of a scientific brotherhood, that resuscitated Vilcek's anti-TNF antibody from its apparent moribund state to become a multibillion-dollar blockbuster,[11] which rapidly changed medical practice, revolutionized the status of rheumatology as a medical discipline, and ushered in a new pharmaceutical era. A key relationship in what became a period of hurtling progress in the development of anti-TNF therapy was that between Jim Woody and the Australian immunologist Marc Feldmann. After medical school, Marc Feldmann earned a PhD in immunology at the Walter and Eliza Hall Institute in Melbourne, Australia, in 1972 with the legendary immunologist Sir Gustav Nossal. Feldmann was an immensely hardworking student, and one day Sir Gus saw firsthand the intensity of that dedication while shopping in a delicatessen in Kew, a suburb of Melbourne. "I met Marc walking towards me along the aisle and propped up in the front of his trolley was a copy of the *Journal of Experimental Medicine* which he was reading with total concentration."[12] Sir Gus freely admits that "Marc was the probably cleverest student I ever had,"[13] and after graduating, Feldmann left Australia to advance his career in the laboratory of world-renowned immunologist Avrion "Av" Mitchison at the Imperial Cancer Research Fund's Tumor Necrosis Unit, before moving to the Kennedy Institute of Rheumatology, London. The beginning of the personal friendship between Jim Woody and Marc Feldmann began in London in the 1980s when Woody, funded by the U.S. Navy, had done research for his PhD under Feldmann's supervision.[14]

During the 1980s and 1990s, the science of immunology came of age with its ability to identify important drug targets for technologists involved in antibody engineering. Leading this wave of identification was the research program designed by Feldmann and his colleague, the Indian-born clinician Sir Ravinder "Tiny" Maini, on the autoimmune disease rheumatoid arthritis. Their collaboration, which began in 1984, formed a milestone in the evolution of our understanding of the mechanism of rheumatoid arthritis through what Woody describes as "the meticulous analysis of genes, tissues, cytokines, and immune responses that led to bone erosion and the fundamental problems of rheumatoid arthritis."[15] One of the most insightful and telling observations made by the team assembled by Feldmann and Maini resulted from an experiment carried out by Fionula Brennan (who tragically died young of breast cancer in 2012).[16] Rheumatoid arthritis (RA) is characterized by a chronic inflammation of the synovial joints and the progressive erosion of cartilage and bone. Brennan's vital contribution was to add the TNF antibody—

that Woody had given to the laboratory—to cells taken from the diseased joints of patients. At the time, it was well known that when cartilage from patients with RA was examined in tissue culture, a whole armada of cytokines, including IL-1, IL-6, IL-8, IL-10, and TNF, were present. What Brennan discovered was that when TNF was blocked, these other cytokines stopped being produced by the cells. According to Jim Woody, this was "a fundamental discovery, and I give Fionula a lot of credit for that."[17] The observation suggested a degree of connectivity between the cytokines and that TNF was at the apex of a proinflammatory "cascade" and, hence, "that blocking TNF might be therapeutically useful in RA."[18] This compelling finding offered Maini, Feldmann, and their team a trial-able hypothesis, which by 1990 they were determined to test.

In translational medicine, the journey between research at the laboratory bench and a drug being used in the clinic is often long, arduous, and frustrating. Indeed, the failure rate is so high—nine times out of ten[19]—that not all scientists want their animal models put to the clinical test.[20] There was no such hesitancy on the part of Feldmann and Maini to seek verification of their hypothesis; indeed, other experienced researchers offered reassurance and encouragement. During one memorable meeting, the influential immunologist James Gowans, who had made significant discoveries about the role of the lymphocyte in the immune response,[21] encouraged Tiny Maini to "go for the jugular"[22] and try the TNF antibody in patients with RA. Having immunologically identified their target, it was decided that Marc Feldmann would call Jim Woody at Centocor to find out if he would be willing to give them enough of the anti-TNF antibody to administer to patients. "So, Marc called me," Woody recalled when we meet some two decades later at Trinity College, Oxford, "and said, 'you know I think this will work in patients,' and my reply was, okay, I will send you enough for a ten-patient trial at something around 10 mg per kilo of antibody."[23] Without this personal connection, it is very possible that Tiny Maini and Marc Feldmann's experiment would have failed to gain traction,[24] because at the time, very few people in the biotech industry believed that the administration of a monoclonal antibody to TNF could be helpful in anything, especially not in a chronic disease where other cytokines were known to be active.

The first ten-patient trial took place at Charing Cross Hospital in London in April 1992, in the form of a small, open (with no placebo control) phase I/II clinical trial under the clinical supervision of Tiny Maini. "It was a safety trial essentially," remembered Tiny Maini when we discussed the path-breaking experiment in 2013. The twenty patients Maini recruited to the trial came from a cohort who had not responded to other treatments for RA. Nevertheless, he was sufficiently worried that nursing care was provided through the night to check on the patients' well-being. Maini feels strongly that this is another aspect of the story that should not go unnoticed: "Without our patient-partners, we couldn't have done this work. They showed a huge amount of trust in allowing us to do something which we couldn't say was completely safe."[25] Not only was it safe, but within a few days,

the condition of all patients treated improved dramatically. The reduced production of TNF and other inflammatory cytokines meant that there was a reduction
in swelling and tenderness in patients' joints and a tangible sense of physical well-
being. "Marc called me the next day," Jim Woody remembered with forensic accuracy, "and he said, 'it is unbelievable, the first thing the patients tell us is that their
pain is gone, and after that they are walking around.'"[26] The improvement was genuine and physiologically verifiable, but unfortunately, the progress proved ephemeral as all of patients relapsed once the treatment had stopped.

Daniel M. Davies, in his insightful and well-conceived book *The Beautiful Cure:
Harnessing Your Body's Natural Defences*, described that this short-lived improvement to the patients' condition indicated to the researchers that obviously, "the
antibody wasn't a cure; but it could relieve symptoms. This meant that the next
logical step was to test the benefits of blocking the cytokine repeatedly."[27] Accordingly, patients were selected in an open-label trial for retreatment by the researchers, and again all of the patients improved, showing that the cA2 antibody may be
effective in the long-term management of the disease.[28] It was then decided to
substitute the observational for the experimental approach through the investigation of the efficacy—or otherwise—of the therapy under the rigorous testing of a
randomized controlled trial. The results of the trial confirmed the earlier findings,
providing "the first good evidence that specific cytokine blockade can be effective
in human inflammatory disease and define a new direction for treatment of rheumatoid arthritis."[29]

Soon, however, a problem was discovered with the chimeric antibody cA2, now
termed infliximab (and marketed as Remicade): it was immunogenic in humans,
because of the mouse content, which caused some patients to make human antichi-
meric antibodies (HACAs) to cA2. Subsequently, Feldmann and Maini devised
a successful way to eliminate this problem by administering a low dose of methotrexate together with the antibody as a combination therapy.[30] This was, according to
Tiny Maini, "a magical combination,"[31] which he later patented with Marc Feldmann.
In the years that followed, the patent had to be vigorously defended in the courts against
the forces of Big Pharma, and according to David Isenberg, a past president of
the British Rheumatology Society, "that patent keeps the Kennedy Institute of
Rheumatology going and also supports Arthritis Research UK."[32] The prodigious
success of Remicade resuscitated the fortunes of Centocor, which was acquired
in 1999 by the multinational pharmaceutical company Johnson & Johnson for
$4.9 billion.[33]

To those who say that the discovery of anti-TNF therapy in the treatment of
RA made by the powerful Maini-Feldmann duumvirate would have inevitably
been achieved by other researchers, this is probably true. Because after all, science
progresses step by incremental step to bring the combined wisdom of many investigators together to add to the great structure of medical knowledge. But what is
equally true is that a unique set of conditions existed in U.K. science in the 1980s
and 1990s that amalgamated and foreshadowed a new era of targeted and highly

effective therapeutics for rheumatoid arthritis and other chronic inflammatory diseases.[34] Moreover, any work that seeks to elucidate the pathogenesis of disease must begin and end with observations in patients, whatever the intermediate steps may be. Thus, indisputably, Marc Feldmann and Tiny Maini's group was the first to take the bold step of treating long-suffering patients with RA with monoclonal antibodies, and their action helped to transform the pharmaceutical landscape.

Where, I hear you ask, is the contribution of Tony Cerami to this extraordinary story of therapeutic advance? It is often the fate of pioneers to be sidelined by history. This is true of the innovative work of Maclyn McCarthy, who in 1944 showed that DNA is the carrier of genes, and Michael Gillies, the medical entomologist and nemesis of malarial mosquitoes—the influence of both of these researchers has been obfuscated by time and the ahistorical influence of restrictive literature reviews that conflate past medical progress with the events of the preceding ten or twenty years. But reparative efforts are being made: in Cerami's case, the Dutch rheumatologist Ferdinand Breedveld, who was one of the leading collaborators in the antibody-methotrexate trial in 1998, is in no doubt of the significance of Cerami to the anti-TNF story: "With Tony Cerami, you have the true genealogy."[35] This point is reinforced by Kevin Tracey, the neurosurgeon who in the 1980s carried out research with Cerami and Beutler on TNF in sepsis and shock: "No Tony Cerami, no anti-TNF. Now, of course you can add other people to that list. You can add Bruce [Beutler], you can add me, you can add Marc [Feldmann], and you can add Tiny [Maini]. But it is clear that Tony was first."[36]

I began this brief overview of the anti-TNF therapy story with the work of basic scientist Jan Vilcek, who is better placed than most to adjudicate the complex interplay between scientific originality, the effect of the expansion of time, and the vicissitudes of the life scientific: "Some consider Lloyd Old the discoverer of TNF, and with good reason, but Tony deserves more recognition for what he did. Unfortunately, I don't think many people know about his work these days—it is now too far in the past."[37] Distance in time is not simply the reason why Cerami's work on TNF has not been remembered: the most enduring contributions came later, with the work of Maini and Feldmann underscoring the collectivist nature of biomedical science while at the same time demonstrating just how arduous the pathway of translational medicine can be on the journey from conceptual breakthrough to use in a clinical setting. Cerami's earlier basic discoveries, however, were the platform upon which these subsequent vital advances were launched.

13 · TAKING ON BIG PHARMA

> The question of being anxious about the future, I'm as anxious as you are, and
> anxiety is something we all have to look forward to.
>
> —Anthony Cerami, speech to Cook College graduates, May 23, 1998

Nineteenth-century philosopher Friedrich Nietzsche famously declared that "there are no facts, only interpretations."[1] This assertion perfectly describes the nuanced context in which lengthy, controversial, and defining court cases involving Cerami took place earlier this century. Opposing lawyers occupied the Nietzschean arena, and their differing interpretations of linguistic understanding and the pliability of language give rare insights into how anti-TNF therapies evolved rapidly to become a $300 billion industry and also offer a highly personalized view of the bitter struggles that have taken place between discovery scientists and the leviathans of the biologics industry. During two major trials, Cerami had his status as a biomedical scientist challenged and his integrity impugned, and he regularly had to bear uncomfortable witness to the ingenious soldering together of disparate fragments of knowledge by adversarial lawyers who believed that they knew what he meant better than he did himself. Of course, Cerami was no stranger to the rebukes and melodramas of the courtroom as over the years he had "made lawyers a lot of money,"[2] but he was now moving into a different dimension in relation to levels of scrutiny, legal costs, and financial settlements of potential transcendental magnitudes.

The astonishingly high profits that were being made by two companies that produced anti-TNF therapies based on the Cerami and Kawakami patents framed the background in which the first lawsuit took place in 2004, in the Eastern District of Texas, for patent infringement. In this case, The Rockefeller University and Chiron Corporation sued Centocor, Inc. and Abbott Laboratories,[3] specifically identifying Remicade and Humira as the respective offending products. At the time, sales of Remicade and Humira had exceeded $3.5 billion and were expected to rise significantly over the next several years. Cerami had been vigilant in protecting his patent rights, orchestrating their renewal when they approached their time-limited duration; furthermore, it was his assiduousness that alerted The Rockefeller University and Chiron that Centocor and Abbott were probably infringing on the patents with their anti-TNF therapies. Throughout the legal process, Cerami attended all of the hearings, providing key scientific advice to The Rockefeller University and Chiron lawyers, and testified for many days on direct and cross-examination.

The trial became notorious for a personal entanglement that was far closer to home when one of the major scientific issues relating to the patent began to be interrogated by a cadre of opposing expert witnesses. The matter in question was whether it was possible to make an antibody to TNF if you did not have a purified protein. The noise of the shuffling of papers and the puffing of cheeks spread among Cerami's supporters when, to their consternation, Bruce Beutler, in a televised deposition, "testified against Tony Cerami."[4] Charles Dinarello was one of the expert witnesses in court that day watching the drama unfold: "Bruce said that Tony was wrong, that you couldn't make an antibody. And this was coming from the guy who purified the molecule!"[5] Dinarello then recommended to The Rockefeller University lawyers to contact his colleague in Boston, Lee Nadler, an expert in monoclonal antibody technology, to oppose Beutler's testimony. Nadler stated that "you do not need a purified protein to make a monoclonal antibody"[6] if you had a good bioassay, which Cerami did, and this evidence according to Dinarello was decisive. "Lee said that Bruce was wrong and Tony won based on Lee opposing Bruce."[7] The motivations responsible for this strange and emotionally charged episode are multilayered, and Dinarello, who has known both Cerami and Beutler for decades, reflects on the underlying dynamics of the scientific schism: "But why would Bruce want to trash Tony on this issue? He used science, he didn't attack him personally. In retrospect, why would Bruce even agree to testify against Tony? That is the bigger question? Why would you? Tony . . . gave him a project that made [his] career: 'here is the project, if you succeed, you'll become famous.' Bruce did become famous, so here's a guy that makes your career, gives you the opportunity, and now you're going to oppose him . . . ? That just looks bad."[8]

After two years of litigation and a favorable ruling on the classification of Cerami's patents, the parties reached separate settlements with the two companies. Centocor settled first. In December 2005, as part of the settlement, the parties entered into a licensing agreement, under which Remicade was a licensed product. In exchange for a quarterly royalty payment to Chiron of 0.75 percent of Remicade's net sales, Centocore obtained a nonexclusive worldwide sublicense to the Cerami patents. A year later, Chiron was acquired by Novartis Vaccines and Diagnostics, Inc. and renamed Novartis. In September 2006, Abbott also settled. The settlement included a covenant not to sue and permitted sales of Humira during the life of the Cerami patents until 2014. The parties agreed Abbott would make a lump-sum payment to be determined by arbitrators. In arbitration, Cerami was Novartis's (formally Chiron) "star witness,"[9] and the arbitrators awarded Novartis $100 million, the highest permissible amount.

The protracted litigation took its toll on Cerami. Masanobu Kawakami, also present at the trial, likewise found cross-examination deeply unsettling, recalling that "my memory of the experience in the court was a terrible one, although a very rare experience in my history. I learned that the psychological stress really causes strong stomach pain, nausea, and vomiting. Before the appearance in court, I thought that the stomach pain, the stress, was a kind of metaphor."[10] As Kawakami and Cerami found out, being cross-examined can be an unnerving and sometimes disturbing experience. If an expert witness cannot be shaken or undermined, then opposing lawyers will try to use a different tactic, possibly looking for vanity, arrogance, or some other weakness in which they can find advantage. As one would expect, the pharmaceutical companies spared no expense on mounting their defense, and consequently, Cerami faced the accusatorial intensity of lawyers whose mastery of the courtroom went beyond the cross-examination technique. Distraction tactics were constantly used, and Cerami's hearing deficit was exploited by lawyers while all of the time the science that underpinned the patents was relentlessly interrogated. A cat-and-mouse game ensued, for instance, over the semantics of discovery:

QUESTION: *Did you identify the mediator in the September 1982 application as TNF?*
ANSWER: No we did not name it TNF.
Q: *Didn't you identify the 70,000 Dalton mouse fraction that is mentioned in the application as cachectin?*
A: As I've told you before, we called it cachectin.
Q: *Did you identify it in the September 1982 application as cachectin?*
A: We didn't give it a name.
Q: *Did you identify the 70,000 Dalton mouse fraction referenced in the September 1982 application as TNF?*
A: We identified a protein which had an apparent molecular weight, 70,000 which had the ability to suppress lipoprotein lipase. A rose is a rose no matter what you call it.
Q: *Can you answer my question?*
A: I did answer your question? You are playing names. I'm not saying its name. I'm saying it's a protein.[11]

Beyond the legal and linguistic tangles of the courtroom, the eroding scrutiny of the trial procedure had revealed unbridgeable fissures between Cerami and The Rockefeller University, the custodian of his scientific discoveries, and, more profoundly, with his former collaborator-employer, Novartis (formally Chiron), who he believed had become unjustly enriched from his scientific insights and intellectual property (IP).[12] What the trial and its many tribulations exposed to Cerami was the duplicitous manner in which Novartis had acted.

In 1985, in the immediate aftermath of Cerami's breakthrough discovery, Chiron had made a formal approach seeking to persuade him to work collaboratively with the company to find ways to commercially exploit his important observations. Step one was to acquire the legal rights to the technology, which under university rules were owned by The Rockefeller University. Chiron achieved that goal by negotiating a license agreement with Rockefeller and their general counsel,

William H. Griesar, in June 1985. At the time, Chiron saw Cerami as a "rising star"[13] of biomedical science and believed that his personal involvement in the venture was so critical to its success that it insisted on negotiating a separate contract with him to better incentivize his focus on their collaborative endeavor. To that end, Chiron's then president, Edward E. Penhoet, drafted a letter confirming the payment of a royalty "of between one-half percent (0.5%) and one percent (1%) of net sales on any products on which Chiron pays a royalty to The Rockefeller University pursuant to the License Agreement, dated June 28 1985, between Chiron and Rockefeller."[14] At no time during the TNF litigation did Novartis state that it would refuse to honor its obligations to Cerami under this 1985 agreement. Nevertheless, following the conclusion of the arbitration in 2006, Novartis steadfastly refused to pay Cerami "at least one half of one percent (0.5%) of the sales of products on which it had paid a royalty to Rockefeller University." Clearly, Novartis believed that Winston Churchill had been correct when he stated that scientists should be "on tap and not on top" in public life and repeatedly rejected Cerami's attempts to have his contract honored. This corporate implacability aroused in Cerami a deep sense of moral indignation. After all, he had fulfilled the undertakings requested of him during the trial only to be denied proper remuneration for his science. Meanwhile, Novartis had secured enormous sums of money and would continue to do so into the future based on Cerami's biomedical discoveries. In truth, Cerami's patents were the cornerstone of a new era in the pharmaceutical industry—the age of "biologic" drugs. Within a very short space of time, anti-TNF therapy had revolutionized the management of many chronic diseases including Crohn's disease, rheumatoid arthritis, and psoriasis. In 1999, when Johnson & Johnson (J&J) acquired Centocor for $4.9 billion, it seemed to be a very generous price given that Centocor's product sales were still modest, but less than a decade later, it was apparent that J&J had got a huge bargain. The success of infliximab paved the way for the development and introduction of other drugs with a similar mechanism of action.[15] All of these drugs (Amgen's Enbrel, UCB's Cimzia, and J&Js Simponi) entered a market that was extremely profitable, growing exponentially, and followed the pharmacological principles of blocking the action of TNF with antibodies.

Indisputably, Cerami too was a beneficiary of the litigation against Centocor and Abbott and shared with his colleague, Masanobu Kawakami, 33 percent of The Rockefeller University's recovery from the settlement, which amounted to the not inconsiderable sum of $8.7 million. Nonetheless, he was adamant that his royalty agreement was a legally binding contract that he had entered into in good faith. Novartis's intransigence appalled him, not only for its dishonesty and its violation of the rules of arithmetic, but self-evidently, within their restricted concept of justice, corporate fealty was more important than contractual loyalty. The disagreement brought into sharp relief the asymmetric balance of power that existed between a biomedical researcher who sought to translate discoveries to find new treatments to treat disease and Big Pharma's overriding purpose to maximize profits.

Dutch rheumatologist Ferdinand Breedveld had become involved in anti-TNF therapy at its inception, playing a major role in a historic randomized controlled trial in 1994.[16] Breedveld sees in Cerami's research the true beginning of TNF's scientific genealogy and can historically contextualize better than most the commercial magnitude of the biologics industry: "There are four companies that dominate the TNF inhibitor market and they have an annual market value of over $30 billion—much of that is profit. And if Tony got a few million it would still be too little for the person who invented it all. That would be unfair."[17] For his part, Cerami was steadfast in his belief that the principles of natural justice had been abandoned by Novartis and that he had successfully delivered "on the excellent scientific achievements" anticipated in Edward E. Penhoet's letter of August 16, 1985. Accordingly, in June 2007, Cerami jettisoned all thoughts of capitulation and instead sued Novartis, a titan of the pharmaceutical industry, over royalty payments in federal court in Manhattan, New York City. In 1985, Novartis had drawn up a contract with Cerami that was designed to incentivize him financially to better focus his attention on their specific biomedical requirements and thereby reduce what was tendentiously observed as a propensity for "wandering to other projects that academics are wont to do."[18] Twenty-two years later, his attention was still fully focused, and he was utterly determined to attain fair remuneration for his scientific contribution to the new multibillion-dollar blockbuster drug class.

Throughout the case presented to the jury in June 2007, the central dispute was over the meaning of two words "any products" in a one-page contract.[19] Explicitly, the disagreement was over what "products" were covered by Novartis's obligation to pay Cerami in connection with *any products* on which Chiron paid a royalty to The Rockefeller University. Cerami insisted that the agreement meant what it said: "any products" means *any* products. Novartis insisted that the contract did not mean what it said. As Novartis's attorneys stated, "Our contention is . . . it was clearly limited to products produced out of the project for sale by Chiron."[20] This was an entirely disingenuous defense, because as a nascent company, Chiron was never in a position to develop its own therapeutics based on capital-intensive recombinant technology. Instead, Chiron Corporation's business plan was to approach big pharmaceutical companies with sublicense proposals and indeed had even gone as far as using Cerami as a scientific emissary to try and secure such a deal with Bayer. For his part, what Cerami sought was royalty payments based on the precedent of monies secured in the infringement litigation, as those products (Remicade and Humira) owed their existence to discoveries he had made at The Rockefeller University.

The two-week-long litigation was a hard-fought exploration of semantics and the subtleties of interpreting what "any products" meant in a contract that had been drafted twenty-two years previously. But to only concentrate on this one, albeit highly significant issue, would underestimate the influence of the other potent contextual layers of meaning that infused the courtroom. Crucially, the case took place in New York, where it was probably true to say that there was not a lot of love for pharmaceutical companies. They were seen as entities that conjured up in people's minds thoughts of the unacceptable face of capitalism, Faustian morality, legions of lawyers, and deep pockets. Adding to the subtext was that just three years before, Cerami had successfully taken on two other pharmaceutical giants and now he appeared before a jury of eight of his peers that would adjudicate between a version of events as told by a lone scientist-inventor or by Big Pharma. "It was," in the opinion of Sharon H. Stern, a member of Cerami's defense team, "a David versus Goliath case, and Tony saw it as a matter of principle, he believed that the drugs that were being produced and sold for vast profits derived from his work."[21] As a witness, Cerami had many attributes, and as the trial unfolded, his character, his focus, and the human and humble manner in which he described his dedication to research, and to finding ways to use science to help sick people, were as affecting as the legal-linguistic interpretations of the two words that dominated proceedings.

Authenticity is everything when a case is taking place in front of a jury, and the arguments and witnesses must come across as credible if a positive outcome is to be forthcoming. It is an arena in which any vulnerability becomes magnified; this added to the already high stakes for which Cerami was playing. If his case was insufficiently persuasive, then the jury was obliged to reject both his financial damages theory and his calculations; such a decision would effectively end his scientific career and endanger his own economic stability.[22] His vulnerability was not lost on the lawyers representing Novartis. The strategy they deployed was an intellectual pincer movement, one arm of which was an undermining of Cerami's character and his science, while the other arm insisted that any monies attained via infringement litigation was to be completely off-limits from the jurisdiction of a poorly drafted contract that did not reflect the complex characteristics of the pharmaceutical industry. The first element of their attack seemed incongruous to the jury, because in the first trial, Cerami had been "practically beatified"[23] by Novartis's (Chiron's) attorneys when they needed him to defend the righteousness of their case, only to have his status reproached with later descriptions of being "unreliable" and that his testimony should be taken with "a considerable grain of salt."[24] The other part of the pincer movement that progressively seemed to ring hollow was the intimation that it was other scientists and not necessarily Cerami who were the progenitors of anti-TNF therapies. Over the course of the trial, the jury began to get a measure of Cerami the man and see at close quarters his tenacity and deep personal commitment to science, as well as his addiction to the excitement and romance of scientific research. And it may well have been this combination of his work and his character that succeeded in disarming the most harmful elements of the Novartis lawyers' protestations. In a court case, as in life, occasionally something happens that seems innocuous but, with the passing of time, takes on greater meaning. Just such an event took place as the trial was coming to an end. Cerami told the jury that he had kept his contract tucked away securely in a safe with other important keepsakes and that he had tried his level best to help companies commercialize his ideas over many decades. This simple story, told in a very matter-of-fact way, seemed, in the opinion of Sharon H. Stern, to ring true with the jury. "Here he was, Dr. Cerami, a world-renowned scientist, but everyone could relate to putting a piece of paper, a book or a letter, something that was important to them, in a safe place." It was a humanizing moment and, for Stern, "made Tony and the jury one."[25]

At the end of the two-week trial, the jury needed just one day to return a verdict in favor of Cerami. Weighing all the facts, the jury unanimously agreed with Cerami's interpretation of the contract and rejected Novartis's. Accordingly, the jury awarded Cerami over $61 million in damages, which, as the parties agreed, was 0.5 percent of net sales through 2008 of Humira and Remicade. With prejudgment interest, the judgment came to $69,432,2337.30. Cerami's personal lawyer, Michael Friedman, who possessed an encyclopedic knowledge of restitutive law, was fond of saying, "When money is involved there's trouble; when big money is involved there's big trouble."[26] The trouble in question came in the form of corporate retaliation when Novartis appealed the judgment and sought a reversal of the jury's verdict, stating that in their opinion, "The district court committed reversible error in directing a verdict on damages."[27] Any sensation that Cerami and his supporters had of floating on the high tide of justice was ended abruptly.

The trial was a decisive moment in Cerami's life because in several ways, it changed his interpretation of the past and altered the trajectory of his future. First, his beloved The Rockefeller University had refused to stand shoulder-to-shoulder with him in the litigation even though he had been their leading expert witness in the earlier successful trial against Centocor and Abbott, which had helped to secure the university a settlement that ran to several tens of millions of dollars. This failure by the university to support his own attempt at obtaining justice was tantamount to abandonment and left him without the institutional support that may have restricted Novartis's relentlessly trenchant litigious zeal. Second, he had put himself through the vicissitudes of the courtroom because he was hugely excited by his discovery of the innate repair receptor (IRR) and the potential to translate this work into new therapies for a variety of diseases, including neuropathy and sarcoidosis. This was the future he envisaged, but he recognized that developing, launching, and commercializing therapies to repair the damage caused by disease would need sums of money that only industrial-sized corporations possessed. Finally, the case can be seen as a turning point in his personal life as the growing disenchantment resulting from a headlong series of failed relationships had finally ended when he married for the fourth time in 2008. His wife, Annie Dunne, a formidable, business-savvy working artist from California, was his consummate cheerleader throughout the entirety of the court cases.[28] He may have had no institutional support from his alma mater, but in "Annie," he had his most ardent, optimistic, and capable supporter. Nothing fired up her sense of injustice more or, in the vernacular of her native La Jolla, "grinds her gears" than intended exploitation. Annie's pushback was instinctive, and if Novartis were determined to appeal the case, then they would be opposed by one of the most distinguished appellate lawyers in the

United States. Josh Rosenkranz, of Orrick, Herrington & Sutcliffe, was retained to handle the appeal, and Cerami's case could not have been in better hands. The *American Lawyer* magazine would later name Rosenkranz "Litigator of the Year" for his professional prowess and even gave him the nomenclature of "the Defibrillator" based on his appellate wins for clients that "appeared at death's door."[29] Novartis signposted the seriousness of their intention to seek a new trial by engaging the formidable Evan R. Chesler of the New York law firm, Cravath, Swaine and Moore. Ordinarily in the United States, only a small fraction of cases in commercial disputes involving pharma companies goes to trial; in fact, over 90 percent of all commercial litigation is settled before reaching a courtroom.[30] But it appeared that Novartis was drawing a line in the sand. While it was true that they had the financial muscle to metabolize failure, they had already incurred significant losses, together with suffering the blunt trauma of adverse publicity in the media.[31] The initial trial had cost Chiron (Novartis) approximately $18 million[32] in legal expenses, and in December 2008, Novartis had paid The Rockefeller University a total of $40,900,919; accordingly, much was at stake for the company. As another trial would burden both Cerami and Novartis with punitive costs, Chesler and Rosenkranz,[33] specialists in commercial dispute resolution, were tasked with finding a settlement that was mutually acceptable and protected by a legally binding confidentiality agreement that prevented Cerami from revealing anything about the negotiated agreement.

The mental and moral toughness that had sustained Cerami throughout the years of litigation continued to strengthen his resolve as he turned his full attention to his latest discovery, TNF's biological antithesis, the innate repair receptor (IRR). Following their unsuccessful business ventures with Lundbeck and Shire, in 2006, Brines and Cerami had founded Araim Pharmaceuticals,[34] which became the vehicle from which they launched the new peptide library of specific ligands designed to activate tissue protection and anti-inflammatory repair. In the short term, the business focus was equally concentrated on Warren and Araim, but as it became increasingly difficult to get business partners to work on carbamylated erythropoietin (cEPO) and the protein portfolio, it was Araim that came to occupy Cerami's attention. The accelerated expansion of Araim Pharmaceutical's scientific program and the corresponding decline of the status of Warren were symptomatic of a change not only in biomedical approach but of a growing partition within the Cerami family. The lightness and excitement of the early years of the Kenneth S. Warren Institute had gone, corrupted in the dirty-air slipstream of Wellstone Filters and Jeremiah Hand's deceptions. As a father, Cerami was generous, critical, humorous, and interested in his children's achievements, but in the laboratory, he could be a passionate autocrat. These competing desires, to be a good father and a wholly committed scientist, came to a thorny apotheosis with his daughter, Carla, when Cerami elected to put all of his efforts into the clinical application of ARA 290 and remove himself entirely from the day-to-day life of the rural laboratory in Westchester County. Here again we witness the flash of a

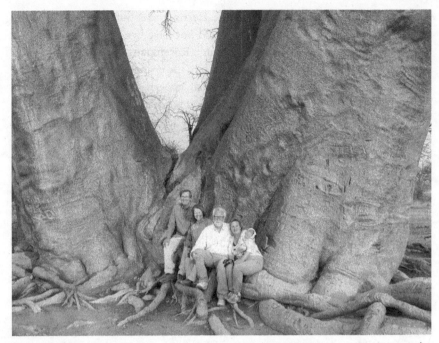

From Mike; "Group at Chapman's Baobob Botswana" (Mike Brines, Pat, Tony, and Annie).

paradox: protective and demanding, the personal warmth that could on occasion be replaced by Antarctic chill cold-shouldering, from needing the close proximity of a community of fellow scientists to being compelled by an equally irresistible force field to move back into solitude. Like a great many creative scientists, or indeed like many of us, Cerami was a complex amalgam of contradictions: with several of his close personal and professional relationships, there was a corresponding excommunication, bridge building followed by bridge burning, and every forward move in science seemed to come at a heavy personal cost. Indeed, at the same time as Cerami made the new biological discovery of the innate repair receptor (IRR), Carla Cerami, an outstanding scientist in her own right,[35] was to recede further from his parental attention with each passing year.

In 1998, Cerami had told students at Rutgers University that "anxiety is something we all have to look forward to"—a decade later, he was understandably feeling anxious about where his future was taking him. It seemed that each brief eureka moment was tempered by years of dedicated and difficult work. But to live an original life of creativity and scientific innovation requires a courageous heart and a thick skin; in 2008, both were tested to their limits and beyond.

Scientifically, there was a still a groundswell of opposition from Big Pharma, in particular Amgen,[36] to the idea that EPO was responsible for any activity other than the promotion of red blood cells. This secular but almost religiously held repudiation of Cerami's work reached its apogee in an article published in *Blood* in 2010.

The multiauthored study stated categorically that "we do not think that clinical studies examining an alleged 'direct' effect of ESAs [erythropoiesis-stimulating agents] on heart or brain function or repair are well founded."[37] This seemed a particularly outlandish statement, as at the time there were multiple labs across the world examining the biological function of the erythropoietin receptor (EPOR). Some of Cerami's likeminded colleagues sought to respond to the published criticisms in the pages of *Blood*, but bearing in mind that the journal was supported financially by Amgen,[38] their right of reply was denied. However, on June 19, 2010, thirty-four researchers, including Cerami, wrote a reply article published in the *Lancet* entitled "Erythropoietin: Not Just about Erythropoiesis," in which they directly addressed what they believed were preconcerted criticisms of their work. The authors were adamant that erythropoietin is active on nonhemopoietic cells and reinforced their finding by stating that "over the past 10 years, multiple investigators have shown that erythropoietin is tissue-protective, anti-inflammatory, and promotes neurogenesis and angiogenesis."[39] The authors concluded their reasoned defense with an allusion to pharma constricting the space in which research takes place: "Although, from a pharmaceutical perspective, it would be convenient if erythropoietin had no activities outside erythropoiesis, this is wishful thinking. The field would be better served by efforts to understand the full spectrum of erythropoietin's actions." This problem of Big Pharma enclosing off areas of research and preventing others from disturbing the status quo was taken up by another pioneer of EPO-protection patents, clinical neuroscientist Hannelore Ehrenreich. In the 1990s, Ehrenreich became acutely interested in the using recombinant human EPO for treatment of stroke and developed an antibody that the nervous system expressed through the EPO receptor.[40] In a multiauthored paper that unequivocally reported that erythropoietin exerts potent neuroprotective functions and called for the development of EPO for therapeutic use outside the hematopoietic system, it also emphasized the inescapable economic mores in which scientific research takes place. "This, in turn, raised discussions within the scientific community, questioning the expression of EPOR in extrahematopoietic tissues. These discussions were likely nurtured by conflicts of interest, trying to restrict the effects of EPO, a highly attractive compound commercially for the anaemia market, to hematopoiesis."[41] All of his scientific life, Cerami had encountered conflicts of interests and the powerful forces of position and opposition, of action and reaction, and now he was determined to break free of the pharmaceutical industry's propensity to thwart his efforts to translate a laboratory discovery into a drug for use in the clinic. But to do this would necessitate moving his center of gravity from the East Coast of the United States to Europe, where he would attempt to establish a series of interlocking collaborations with clinicians and laboratory scientists who were looking for a new healing agent to accelerate the restoration of damaged tissue.

In 2008, to aid his intercontinental transition, Cerami was awarded a prestigious Boerhaave Professorship at the Leiden University Medical Center, Holland.[42]

Once the almost inevitable early difficulties of moving to a new country had been overcome,[43] Leiden, the birth place of Rembrandt, with its centuries-old architecture, civic pride, and effervescent medical school, provided a rich canvas upon which Cerami could portray the biological underpinnings of his innate repair receptor in both health and disease. In his first Boerhaave lecture, Cerami's description of how his 11–amino acid peptide activates the body's natural repair system struck a resonant chord with one member of the audience, Albert Dahan, head of anesthesia and pain research at Leiden University Medical Center. After the lecture, Dahan gathered his postdocs together, telling them that "this drug would work fantastically well in all of these neuropathic pain syndromes that we are looking"[44] because his team believed that neuropathic pain was a form of inflammation. This common ground shaped the basis for a far-reaching collaboration between Araim and Dahan and his colleagues,[45] which moved into clinical research to test the efficacy of ARA 290 to treat neuropathic pain in two chronic diseases: the orphan disease sarcoidosis[46] and type 2 diabetes. Dahan's team progressed along two parallel lines of approach: animal experiments on mice and rats and small randomized controlled trials in patients. "In the animal studies," Dahan enthusiastically recalled, "we understood how Tony's nerve drug ARA 290 started to work and which receptors were activated and we found it mind-blowing. ARA 290 is a very powerful drug, and without Tony, we would not have been on that track, we would still be on the track of opioids."[47]

Within a few years, the peptide, which activates the body's natural repair mechanism, had been tested in many animal models, including head trauma, myocardial infarction, retinal damage, and nerve damage, showing efficacy in stopping inflammation and initiating repair in every tissue evaluated.[48] These findings created fertile ground for further collaborations with scientists across Europe. Uppermost in the minds of Brines and Cerami was to attract "key opinion leaders"[49] to take up their peptide and use it to produce evidence of cellular and tissue repair in various diseases. To this end, Cerami contacted Chris Thiemermann, a pharmacologist and renowned translational scientist at Barts NHS Trust, London. Crucially, Thiemermann had trained with Nobel laureate John Vane, who, like Cerami, was a shrewd and commercially minded scientist. In 2003, Thiemermann had become CEO of William Harvey Research Limited (WHRL), a commercial entity originally created to make links between academic and the pharmaceutical industry—and this was just the vehicle that Cerami was looking to use as a platform for ARA 290, Araim's erythropoietin analogue. Thiemermann and his team were aware of Cerami's article showing that erythropoietin protects the brain, and they were excited about establishing a collaborative relationship to look at the effect of the peptide on the kidney. "We found it highly effective against various insults against the kidney," recalled Thiemermann, "and we started to cooperate on a non-commercial basis, and published a series of studies together."[50]

Cerami's aim had been to get ARA 290 into clinical medicine in diabetes, but Araim could not fund the large randomized controlled trials that the Food and

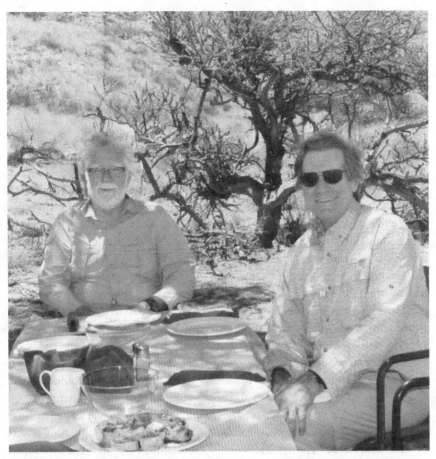

Tony Cerami and his long-time collaborator Mike Brines on holiday in Namibia in 2016.

Drug Administration (FDA) required to satisfy their standards of efficacy and safety. Nevertheless, evidence presented in the academic literature was attracting researchers in the diabetes field. One person at the forefront of diabetes care, and interested in the anti-inflammatory effect of ARA 290, was Swedish endocrinologist Claes-Goran Ostenson, who worked at the Karolinska Institute in Stockholm, Sweden. At the time, Ostenson was working on type 2 diabetes, and while it was known that there was inflammation in the pancreatic islets producing insulin, no one fully understood the mechanism behind this phenomenon. This physiological conundrum gave Ostenson the idea of asking Cerami if it would be possible to conduct a collaborative study; fortuitously, he had developed a very good animal (rat) model of spontaneous type 2 diabetes that might provide some answers.[51] With Cerami's cooperation, Ostenson's team conducted both islet studies and in vivo studies in the hope of gaining a better understanding of basic mechanisms. "We did two things," Ostenson remembered with forensic accuracy, "we isolated the islet, and we took out the pancreas. There was poor secretion without ARA 290, but when we added the peptide, it had fantastic effects, it restored metabolism in the islets."[52] Araim capitalized on the growing body of persuasive research evidence and in 2016 succeeded in persuading the FDA to grant Orphan Drug Designation to ARA 290 for treatment to increase survival and improve the functioning of pancreatic islets following transplantation.

One advantage of having orphan disease status is that the pathway is easier to commercialize, but even so, after twenty years of concentrated work developing an extensive peptide library and having achieved in vivo proof-of-concept efficacy together with an acknowledged legitimacy in the scientific literature, Cerami still did not have a drug approved for use in patients suffering from a major disease. This failure is in part explained by recognizing that the path of scientific discovery from embryonic idea to approved treatment must navigate a number of almost insurmountable hurdles. Preeminently, pharmaceutical companies are very risk averse and will only take on the huge development costs of a drug if effectiveness and safety have been unequivocally proven by large, expensive, randomized controlled trials.[53] As most freestanding laboratories do not have the resources to fund large and increasingly complex clinical trials, this effectively ends the translational journey for a new therapeutic category. Moreover, because ARA 290 is a peptide, with a half-life of only two minutes before it disappears from the body, this ephemeral biological activity aroused skepticism early on that never fully disappeared.[54] This problem of acceptance, as Chris Thiemermann acknowledged, was because "people don't like peptides, they like to know the mechanism, even though we still don't fully understand how aspirin works."[55] But Cerami and Brines were convinced of the molecular mechanisms underlying the long-lasting effects of their short-lived peptide, that it could successfully turn on the innate repair receptor in the same way that one turns on a light switch, and that the activity stayed on for a number of days; however, they were also conscious that the uniqueness of their approach evoked thoughts of "this is all imaginary stuff" in the minds of the key opinion leaders they most wanted convince.[56]

As a means of diluting pharmaceutical companies' skepticism, Cerami spent over $3 million proving that his peptide, which was renamed *cibinetide* (a generic USAN name) in 2016, was not carcinogenic. He had always known that to translate an idea into a possible treatment required a big investment in time, energy, and money, but after all of his efforts, even presenting positive evidence from clinical trials was not enough and perhaps might never be enough.[57] He was conscious that he was caught in a business–biology Catch-22 paradox, and he was not alone; researchers continually discover new biological processes that could be drug targets for major clinical indicators, but these targets are not adequately confirmed to persuade the pharmaceutical industry to enter them into the development process.[58] Increasingly, Cerami felt anxious and discouraged, captive in his own Yossarian-like dilemma—compelled to go forward, as retreat was unthinkable.

In this sense, the episode was the very embodiment of both the complex nature of translational medicine and the possible future direction of drug discovery. One of the most important questions facing medical science is where new drugs are going to come from. Will enlightened empiricism, disease-focused rational drug design, or indeed a combination of both provide some of the answers? Will a fundamental change in the ecosystem of the pharmaceutical industry take place to enable the demarcation lines between industry and academia to dissolve, thereby increasing innovation, reducing wasteful replication, and providing the resources necessary to train the next generation of scientists to work productively on behalf of society?[59] In the case of Cerami's long-standing work on cibinetide, stuck between a product that he wholeheartedly believes in and a pharmaceutical world too reluctant to invest sufficient capital in backing the drug, the immediate solution has been for Cerami to prop up the venture with his own private funding. The future of the drug remains potentially beguiling, yet vulnerable.

Besides his work on ARA 290, Cerami's later years have been diverse and productive. In 2010, Cerami and his wife, Annie, had established a foundation, the Anthony Cerami and Ann Dunne Foundation for World Health, an organization devoted to leading-edge medical research, education, and care. The foundation was a vindication of their shared ideas, and it gave Cerami the opportunity to put his newfound wealth to good use. One of the first medical projects funded by the foundation was a study of thalassemia being carried out by his great friend from the Great Neglected Diseases days, Sir David Weatherall. The joint program between Oxford University and hospitals in Sri Lanka provided a better understanding of the evolutionary biology of the alpha and beta thalassemias and how these disorders might be better controlled or prevented. Although Weatherall was a giant in the field of molecular medicine and had won the Lasker Prize in 2010 for his contribution to clinical medicine, he had found it increasingly difficult to secure grants once he had passed the official retirement age, and this new funding stream allowed him to complete his final medical study in Asia.

Gradually, formal retirement beckoned, and Cerami spent less time in his natural habitat—the lab. But his retirement did not mark an end to his downstream influence on translational medicine or the distinct scientific attitude that he had championed. In the spring of 2018, friends and colleagues of Anthony Cerami gathered in the dazzling location of St. Paul's Church, Frankfurt, Germany, to see him being awarded the Paul Ehrlich and Ludwig Darmstaedter Prize in recognition of his work in the field of cytokine biology and its translation into treatments of TNF-mediated diseases. Since childhood, Ehrlich had been his inspiration, and in a tangential way, it was through Ehrlich's influence that he came to discover TNF; when he got his first Great Neglected Diseases grant from Ken Warren, it was used to work on trypanosomiasis, which his scientific hero had studied a century before. As Cerami walked along the building's imposing marbled floor to give his acceptance speech, he was transported back in time to his childhood when he had read Paul de Kruif's *Microbe Hunters* and the laudatory chapter on Ehrlich entitled "The Magic Bullet." Holding the lectern firmly in both hands, he thought of his own life as a scientist and was reminded of how Ehrlich had skillfully deflected the adulation of a colleague who wanted to portray the discovery of the first medical treatment for syphilis as the work of a great mind and a wonderful scientific achievement. "My dear colleague," said Paul Ehrlich, "for seven years of misfortune I had one moment of good luck."[60]

Like Ehrlich, Cerami's scientific life has been a fusion of luck, misfortune, opportunity, failure, and achievement. The translational approach was for him both an art and a science; the objective was to try to understand the biological pathway of a disease and the course the illness takes in individual patients. To achieve this aim, he focused on work with a synthesized team of investigators—a laboratory without walls—with expertise in chemistry, biology, and medicine to approach diseases from a panorama of perspectives and at different levels. This drive to help people not only satisfied his thirst for discovery but also enabled him to create the conditions in which others could flourish. More than recognition, he wanted to be useful, and he saw his role as providing the connective tissue between scientific insights, understanding diseases, and developing drugs to treat them. This outlook very much conforms to the principles of the translational ethos, a practice gradually evolving during Cerami's working life and continuing to develop in recent years. Indeed, the field of translation has changed significantly over the past half century or more. In the United States in the 1960s, for example, the concept of the triple-threat approach evolved as the ideal of the academic physician. This Edenic vision presupposed that the supercharged individual would be able to (a) perform original primary research, (b) train medical students and residents, and (c) provide high-quality clinical care.[61] But even sixty years ago, this "three-legged stool" archetype may only have existed somewhere between a wonderful hope and myth,[62] while today, the ever increasing growth of specialization and the gap between basic science and clinical medicine can hinder the progression of translation. Another reason, often voiced, as an explanation why drug discovery is becoming more difficult is that the easy targets have largely been solved and that it gets harder to find new treatments for the more challenging diseases.[63] What is less questionable, and which certainly overwhelmingly affected Cerami's life in translation, was that potential partners became increasingly more risk averse, and with each passing decade, the requirements for getting an idea into development changed from merely needing some unsophisticated preclinical data to a demand for persuasive evidence generated by complex and expensive clinical trials. Undeniably, development costs for pharmaceutical companies are high, and findings from a recent study suggested that the average cost of a new drug in the United States is $2.6 billion, up 145 percent in the past decade. These are striking statistics, especially when one remembers that most drug candidates fail.[64] This reality presents researchers with a dichotomy: while the translation of life sciences into therapeutic applications is much in vogue, the macroeconomics that determine this discovery process are virtually insurmountable.

And what of the current crisis that threatens global public health? COVID-19 has led to conventional levels of health spending being held in suspended animation as the vast resources of the world's leading economies are repurposed to find ways to combat an infectious disease. Translational medicine may well mean different things to different people, but in the age of COVID-19, it is now important to us all: the global pandemic has brought the question of how to discover drug treatments and how to translate them from the laboratory to use in potentially billions of people front and center in ways that could never have been imagined just a few years previously. This unprecedented moment places the template of rational drug design that evolved under Cerami's stewardship as the scientific technique at the forefront of attempts by researchers across the world to translate disease-targeted knowledge into treatments on a global scale. This, in turn, raises a multitude of questions surrounding production, distribution, equity, intellectual property, and cost-effectiveness. Cerami's own experiences in translation suggest that the lengthy timeline of potential discovery, its economic costs, and the often fraught but necessary collaborative work between Big Pharma, governments, and public and private institutions are all notes of caution that must be anticipated or resolved if COVID-19 is to be brought under control in a clinical fashion.

For researchers in molecular medicine, investigators pursuing basic science in the hope of improving human health, and indeed anyone seeking to achieve goals in life, much inspiration can be found in the life scientific of Anthony Cerami. His audacious attitude is the crystallization of discovery science at its best: the process of identifying the new, the unknown, and the unexpected while maintaining an eye for the expendable to allow continued dynamic research. This said, Cerami possessed certain inherent and exceptional characteristics that set him apart from other biomedical investigators. His childhood on the family farm coincided with the introduction of antibiotics and chemotherapeutic agents into livestock production and animal feeds.[65] This opened his mind to the idea that the epidemic scourges that only a few months before had frequently annihilated entire populations of his domestic animals could be largely controlled and even eradicated. During these formative years, he also became progressively aware of the devastating burden that diabetes and its complications were having on members of his immediate family. These experiences left a powerful impression because they showed him the relevance of science to solving the problems of daily life, and importantly, they shaped the direction of his subsequent activities. By understanding the fluid interaction between how the broader history of the time in which Cerami lived shaped his ideas and how he in turn imprinted his scientific philosophy on translational science, valuable insights can be found into the future direction of drug discovery.

Cerami's strengths as a scientist were his curiosity, his imagination, and the ability to see patterns and propagate theories. Moreover, he had the capacity to bring together different fields to give new insights into disease processes, while at the same time, and throughout his fifty-year career, he surrounded himself with some of the world's leading scientific intellects who were equally dedicated to translating scientific discoveries into new treatments for patients. Considering how imaginative his ideas were, it is surely not too much to suggest that clinical medicine would not be the same today if it had not been for Cerami; his contributions to the field of diabetes and inflammatory diseases have both reduced the burden of disease and increased human well-being. In relation to diabetes, he was in the vanguard of translational thinking and invented the HbA1c test as an invaluable index of glycemic control. Meanwhile, it is almost certainly true that if Centocor had focused its original efforts on rheumatoid arthritis and not on sepsis—Cerami fought hard against the clinical trial in sepsis because he thought that the disease was too variable in timing and severity—then the clinical application of anti-TNF would have occurred earlier. That it did at all was due in no small part to Cerami's early stage work on TNF at a basic science level. These two gigantic contributions to the medical armamentarium could not have happened without Cerami's vision for turning biological discoveries into diagnostics and medicines. As one former collaborator summarized, "No Tony Cerami, no anti-TNF. No Tony Cerami, no hemoglobin A1c."[66]

Complementing these two giant successes in clinical medicine, Cerami also developed the advanced glycation end products (AGEs) and the protein cross-linking concepts that helped to explain the origin of diabetic complications. His work on AGEs has contributed significantly to the sheer momentum that modern studies of biological aging have gained. Finally, his last and most enduring scientific collaboration was with Mike Brines; their twenty-year partnership developed the innate repair receptor (IRR) and engineered peptides to activate it that are currently in clinical trials. If approved for patients, the lead compound cibinetide has the potential to treat complications of diabetes, with likely far-reaching scientific and commercial implications. This biology also offers the real possibility of clinical translation in the areas of wound healing, transplantation, and neuropathy. In this sense, although the impact of Anthony Cerami's translational science on human health is already profound, it may well increase with the passing of time.

Cerami sees translational science as a principled endeavor that demands intellectual rigor, persistence, devotion, and considerable sacrifice to produce even the most rudimentary insights into the laws of nature. By advocating targeted research on specific diseases, Cerami's approach continues to have an impact on health outcomes. In 1967, when Detlev Bronk spoke in support of Anthony Cerami's candidacy for doctor of philosophy at The Rockefeller University's Convocation for Conferring Degrees, he made a prophetic observation: "Cerami's work has always been pursued with intensity, imagination, sophistication and skill. Because he was always generous and helpful, and willing to share his experiences, he engaged in numerous related collaborative and cooperative undertakings with colleagues in his own and other laboratories ... Cerami is especially well-suited for life at the frontier represented by science. His unusual tenacity and productiveness are driven by a deep personal commitment to science and he has a well-developed taste for the adventure, excitement and romance which are the most attractive elements of scientific research. His scientific efforts will be a credit to science, to himself and to this institution."[67]

Cerami's name may not have obtained the heightened renown of other contemporary medical investigators, but his research, creative leadership, and scientific convening skills have formed the bedrock of translational medicine, without which a generation of subsequent researchers could not have moved forward. What set him apart from other scientists was his extraordinary diversity, which allowed him to cover so much ground,[68] and what followed was a matter of good fortune and providence. At the end of his professional career, Cerami fought against self-delusion every bit as hard as he had done when he was at The Rockefeller University. Above all, he knew what he had done in his scientific and personal life, and just as significantly, he was aware of what he had not be able to achieve. For any of us brave enough to honestly attempt to "know thyself," how we measure our contribution must surely fall within those two compass points of life.

ACKNOWLEDGMENTS

This book began life almost a decade ago when I had the idea to write about one of the most important discoveries in immunological and molecular medicine—that under certain conditions, the human body was capable of attacking itself by the release of the proinflammatory cytokine, tumor necrosis factor (TNF), and that the autoimmune diseases caused by this process could be treated with monoclonal antibodies. This was a discovery that came to be regarded as a decisive moment in modern medicine and launched the new and highly profitable era of anti-TNF biological drugs at the end the twentieth century. However, after a year and many failed attempts to interest U.K. publishers in a story that changed medical practice, I became resolved to the fact that the appetite for biomedical science had declined, and while my commitment to the project remained undiminished, I would be compelled to wait until trends changed before I could take the idea further. Fortuitously, in 2013, my ongoing research led to a meeting with the pathologist Siamon Gordon, a world-renowned expert on macrophages, the family of white blood cells of the immune system that engulf and digest cancer cells and the other foreign matter that might harm the healthy cells of the human body. As soon as Gordon realized that I wanted to write a book about the medical history of TNF and the emergence of translational medicine, he completely transformed the book from being a comprehensive history of an idea into a study of a life when he commented, "You can't write about TNF without knowing about the work of Tony Cerami. We were at The Rockefeller University together in the 1970s; we're still friends and you really should know more about his research." He of course was right, and my subsequent meeting with Anthony Cerami marked the beginning of this biographical study, which has enabled me to write a wider history of the contributions made to the TNF story and to intimately navigate the world of translational medicine by exploring the life of one of the discipline's most influential pioneers.

I owe debts of gratitude to many people, and it is with great pleasure that I thank those who have helped me in the research and writing of *Anthony Cerami: A Life in Translational Medicine*. During the years while working on the book, I have changed my center of gravity, moving from my role of writer-in-residence at The Wellcome Unit for the History of Medicine at Oxford University to a visiting professorship within the School of Medicine at Trinity College Dublin. Consequently, the book forms an important intellectual bridge, linking my decade-long association with colleagues in Oxford and my new career within the vibrant atmosphere of Trinity College. Colleagues in both universities offered innumerable suggestions, ideas, insights, and references that have been incorporated into the book.

During the epic journey of researching this biography, I have interviewed many people too numerous to list individually, but I do want to thank some whose conversations over the years have provided particularly invaluable insights. They include John David, Dan Rifkin, Barbara Sherry, Richard Bucala, Alan Fairlamb, Kevin Tracey, Carol Rouser, Michael Brownlee, Joseph Graziano, Steven Meshnick, Ron Koenig, and many, many others. I benefited greatly from being able to have as my scientific mentor Sir David Weatherall. Alas, David died in December 2018, but those regular meetings in the café of the Weatherall Institute of Molecular Medicine where I would go for help and advice will live long in my memory. Often, David would be sheltering outside his eponymous institute having a few puffs on his pipe to steady his resolve before our work began. Of course, it would have been difficult to write this book without the encouragement and generosity of Mike Brines, and I thank him for his unfaltering enthusiasm for the project. Throughout the research and writing process, I have also enjoyed the support of Annie Dunne, for whom nothing was too much trouble, and numerous boxes of personal papers, scientific notebooks, and photographic albums were dispatched from California and New York to my office in Dublin. Above all, I want to thank Tony Cerami for his full cooperation in telling the story of his life in science, even though he knew it would uncover some uncomfortable truths.

All books need a good editor, and Peter Mickulas at Rutgers University Press was ever helpful. Equally skilled in the use of sticks and carrots, his dedication to detail gave this book a cohesion that it previously lacked. Also deserving of my special appreciation at Rutgers is Karen Li, who did an outstanding job of ensuring stylistic consistency in bringing the book together.

Of course, any mistakes and errors of emphasis, fact, and logic that readers uncover are entirely of my own making.

Conrad Keating
Trinity College Dublin
September 2020

NOTES

FOREWORD

1. P. Hotez, "The Medical Biochemistry of Poverty and Neglect," *Molecular Medicine* 20 (2014): S31–S36; P. Hotez, *Vaccines Did Not Cause Rachel's Autism: My Journey as a Vaccine Scientist, Pediatrician and Autism Dad* (Baltimore: Johns Hopkins University Press, 2018).

INTRODUCTION

1. Interview with Anthony Cerami, June 2018.
2. Interview with William Campbell, May 2016. Campbell is one of the method's foremost exponents and winner of the Nobel Prize in 2015 for his role in discovering ivermectin.
3. C. Monaco, J. Nanchahals, P. Taylor, and M. Feldmann, "Anti-TNF therapy: Past, Present and Future," *International Immunology* 27, no. 1 (January 2015): 55–62.
4. J. Karp and R. McCaffrey, "New Avenues of Translational Research in Leukemia and Lymphoma: Outgrowth of a Leukemia Society of America—National Cancer Institute Workshop," *Journal of the National Cancer Institute* 86, no. 16 (1994): 1196–201.
5. *Essentials for Discovery* (New York: The Rockefeller University, 1984), 8.
6. For more on physician-scientists and a good overview of the topic, see D. Weatherall, *Science and the Quiet Art: Medical Research and Patient Care* (Oxford: Oxford University Press, 1995).
7. G. Mitchell, "Comments on the GND Program," in *The Great Neglected Diseases of Mankind Biomedical Research Network: 1978–1988*, ed. K. Warren and C. Jimenez (New York: The Rockefeller Foundation, 1988), 49.
8. J. Watson and F. Crick, "Molecular Structure of Nucleic Acids: A Structure for Deoxyribose Nucleic Acid," *Nature* 171 (1953): 737–38. For more on the history of molecular biology, see H. Freeland Judson, *The Eighth Day of Creation: Makers of the Revolution in Biology* (Cold Spring Harbor, NY: Cold Spring Harbor Laboratory Press, 1996); G. Hunter, *Vital Forces: The Discovery of the Molecular Basis of Life* (London: Academic Press, 2000); K. Lily, *The Molecular Vision of Life: Caltech, the Rockefeller Foundation and the Rise of the New Biology* (Oxford: Oxford University Press, 1996).
9. Weatherall, *Science and the Quiet Art*, 228.
10. S. Woolf, "The Meaning of Translational Research and Why It Matters," *Journal of the American Medical Association* 299, no. 2 (2008): 211–13.
11. M. Day, "MRC Wants to Cut Time from Bench to Bedside," *British Medical Journal* 334 (2007): 493.
12. Interview with Chas Bountra, May 4, 2020.
13. Interview with Chas Bountra, May 4, 2020.
14. V. McElheny, *Drawing the Map of Life: Inside the Human Genome* (New York: Basic Books, 2010).
15. M. Kawakami, "Discovery of Tumor Necrosis Factor (TNF) and Identification of the Potential of Anti-TNF Antibodies in Dr. Cerami's Laboratory," *Molecular Medicine* 20 (2014): S17–S19.
16. G. Ferry, "Sir Aaron Klug" [obituary], *The Guardian*, November 26, 2018.

1. HARD WORK

1. Interview with Elliott West, November 2017.
2. Interview with Anthony Cerami, May 2016.

3. J. Tarver "Costs of Rearing Farm Children," *Journal of Farm Economics* 38, no. 1 (February 1956): 144–53.

4. O. Baker, "Rural-Urban Migration and the National Welfare," *Annals of the Association of American Geographers* 23, no. 2 (1933): 86–87; O. Baker, *Two Trends of Great Agricultural Significance* (Washington, DC: U.S. Department of Agriculture, Extension Service Circular O. 306, 1939), 6.

5. Tarver, "Costs of Rearing Farm Children," 152.

6. A. Cerami, "GND Note," in *The Great Neglected Diseases of Mankind Biomedical Research Network: 1978–1988*, ed. K. S. Warren & C. C. Jimenez (New York: The Rockefeller Foundation, 1988), 119.

7. A. Cerami, "A Forty-Year Odyssey in the Sea of Translational Medicine," *Proceedings of the American Philosophical Society* 158, no. 4 (December 2014): 408.

8. Clubs were the foundation of the 4-H program—and the name came from the pledge taken by its members: "I pledge my Head to clear thinking, My Heart to greater loyalty, My Hands to larger service, My Health for better living. For my club, my community, my country and my world. I believe in 4-H work for the opportunity it will give me to become a useful citizen." The 4-H slogan is "Learn by doing."

9. J. P. Verhave, "Paul de Kruif: A Michigan Leader in Public Health," *Michigan Historical Review* 39, no. 1 (Spring 2013): 41–69.

10. Anthony Cerami's sister, Judith, also graduated with a bachelor's degree from Barnard College, part of Columbia University.

2. THE ROCKEFELLER EFFECT

1. A. Cerami, "A Surprising Journey in Translational Medicine," *Molecular Medicine* 20 (2014): S2.

2. Interview with Anthony Cerami, June 2016.

3. The Nobel Prize in Physiology and Medicine in 2015 was shared between William Campbell and Satoshi Omura, as well as the Chinese researcher Tu Youyou, for the discovery of artemisinin, a highly effective antimalarial drug now used to treat millions of people every year.

4. J. Cairns, *Matters of Life and Death: Perspectives on Public Health, Molecular Biology, Cancer, and the Prospects for the Human Race* (Princeton, NJ: Princeton University Press, 1997), xi.

5. Interview with Anthony Cerami, June 2016.

6. V. Monnier, R. Kohn, and A. Cerami, "Accelerated Age-Related Browning of Human Collagen in Diabetes Mellitus," *Proceedings of the National Academy of Sciences of the United States of America* 81, no. 2 (January 1984): 583–87.

7. D. H. Stapleton, ed., *Creating a Tradition of Biomedical Research: Contributions to the History of The Rockefeller University* (New York: The Rockefeller University Press, 2004), 5.

8. Stapleton.

9. Interview with Anthony Cerami, June 2016.

10. P. Rous, "Simon Flexner 1863–1946," *Obituary Notices of Fellows of the Royal Society* 6, no. 18 (1949): 408–26.

11. B. Webster, "Dr. Detlev W. Bronk, 78, Of Rockefeller U., Is Dead" [obituary], *New York Times*, November 18, 1975.

12. J. Rogers Hollingsworth, "Institutionalizing Excellence in Biomedical Research: The Case of The Rockefeller University" in Stapleton, *Creating a Tradition of Biomedical Research*, 45.

13. C. P. Snow, Rede Lecture, May 7, 1959.

14. "Minutes of the Rockefeller University Trustees," May 22, 1961, Rockefeller University Archives, in Rogers Hollingsworth, "Institutionalizing Excellence," 42.

15. Rogers Hollingsworth, "Institutionalizing Excellence," 42.

16. Hollingsworth, 43.

17. Interview with Anthony Cerami, June 2016.

18. Interview with Anthony Cerami, June 2016.

19. Cerami, "Surprising Journey," S2.

20. Interview with Anthony Cerami, June 2016.

21. Webster, "Dr. Detlev W. Bronk."

22. Interview with Anthony Cerami, June 2016.

23. Cerami, "Surprising Journey," S3.

24. T. S. Kuhn, *The Structure of Scientific Revolutions* (Chicago: University of Chicago Press, 1962), 36.

25. Interview with Daniel Rifkin, October 2017.

3. THE SHAPING OF A SCIENTIFIC MIND

1. J. Rogers Hollingsworth, "Institutionalizing Excellence in Biomedical Research: The Case of The Rockefeller University," in *Creating a Tradition of Biomedical Research: Contributions to the History of The Rockefeller University*, ed. D. H. Stapleton (New York: The Rockefeller University Press, 2004), 17.

2. J. Butler, H. Romney, and F. Wolling, eds., *The Rockefeller Foundation 1913–1988* (New York: The Rockefeller Foundation, 1989), 3.

3. R. Bremner, *American Philanthropy* (Chicago: Chicago University Press, 1960), 117.

4. Butler et al., *The Rockefeller Foundation 1913–1988*, 4.

5. P. Rosenfield, *A World of Giving: Carnegie Corporation of New York–A Century of International Philanthropy* (New York: Public Affairs, 2014), 38.

6. D. H. Stapleton, "The Rockefeller (University) Effect: A Phenomenon in Biomedical Science," in Stapleton, *Creating a Tradition of Biomedical Research*, 7.

7. https://www.rockefeller.edu/events-and-lectures/facilities-inside/ (accessed April 24, 2018).

8. Interview with Daniel Rifkin, October 2017.

9. Interview with Miki Rifkin, March 2018.

10. The 1958 Nobel Prize in Physiology or Medicine was awarded one half to George Wells Beadle and Edward Tatum "for their discovery that genes act by regulating definite chemical events" and the other half to Joshua Lederberg "for his discoveries concerning genetic recombination and the organization of the genetic material of bacteria." Lederberg was the fifth president of The Rockefeller University, serving from 1978 to 1990.

11. Interview with Edward Reich, May 2016.

12. A. Cerami, E. Reich, D. Ward, and I. Goldberg, "The Interaction of Actinomycin with DNA: Requirement for the 2-Amino Group of Purines," *Proceedings of the National Association of the Academy of Sciences of the United States of America* 57, no. 4 (1967): 1036–42.

13. Interview with Edward Reich, May 2016.

14. Interview with Edward Reich, May 2016.

15. Interview with Edward Reich, May 2016.

16. D. Weatherall, *Science and the Quiet Art: Medical Research and Patient Care* (Oxford: Oxford University Press, 1995), 56.

17. J. Cairns, *Matters of Life and Death: Perspectives on Public Health, Molecular Biology, Cancer, and the Prospects for the Human Race* (Princeton, NJ: Princeton University Press, 1997), 51.

18. Interview with David Ward, January 2018.

19. D. Ward, A. Cerami, E. Reich, G. Acs, and L. Altwerger, "Biochemical Studies of the Nucleoside Analogue, Formycin," *Journal of Biological Chemistry* 244, no. 12 (1969): 3243–50.

20. R. Klett, A. Cerami, and E. Reich, "Exonuclease VI, a New Nuclease Activity Associated with *E. coli* DNA Polymerase," *Proceedings of the National Academy of Sciences of the United States of America* 60, no. 3 (1968): 943–50.

21. Interview with Anthony Cerami, June 2018.

22. Interview with David Ward, January 2018.

23. Interview with David Ward, January 2018.

24. Interview with David Ward, January 2018.

25. Interview with George Cross, March 2018.

26. B. Ehrenreich, *Living with a Wild God: A Nonbeliever's Search for the Truth about Everything* (London: Granta Books, 2014), 170.

27. Ehrenreich, 170.

28. Interview with Miki Rifkin, March 2018.

29. Interview with Miki Rifkin, March 2018.

30. A. Bloom and W. Breines, eds., *Takin' It to the Streets: A Sixties Reader* (New York: Oxford University Press, 1995), 14.

31. Ehrenreich, *Living with a Wild God*, 185.

32. Interview with Anthony Cerami, June 2016.

33. Interview with Siamon Gordon, January 2016.

34. Rogers Hollingsworth, "Institutionalizing Excellence," 31.

35. "Obituary Notice," *The Independent*, October 22, 2008.

36. Interview with Anthony Cerami, June 2016.

37. P. de Kruif, *The Sweeping Wind: A Memoir* (London: Rupert Hart-Davis, 1962), 56.

38. Interview with Siamon Gordon, January 2016.

39. Interview with Alan Kapuler, June 2016.

40. A. Cerami, "A Surprising Journey in Translational Medicine," *Molecular Medicine* 20 (2014): S3.

41. Interview with Alan Kapuler, June 2016.

42. Interview with David Ward, January 2016.

43. S. Greenberg, "Microbe Hunters Revisited—Paul de Kruif and the Beginning of Popular Science Writing," *Houston History of Medicine Lectures*, March 7, 2001, 4.

44. Interview with David Ward, January 2016.

45. Cerami et al., "The Interaction of Actinomycin," 1036–42.

46. Interview with Irving Goldberg, May 2016.

47. Cerami, "Surprising Journey," S3.

48. Interview with Siamon Gordon, January 2016.

49. D. Duncan, *The Life and Letters of Herbert Spencer* (Cambridge: Cambridge University Press, 2014), 513.

50. The Nobel Prize in Physiology or Medicine in 1980 was awarded jointly to Baruj Benacerraf, Jean Dausset, and George D. Snell "for their discoveries concerning genetically determined structures on the cell surface that regulate immunological reaction."

51. D. Coleman and K. Hummel, "Studies with the Mutation, Diabetes, in the Mouse," *Diabetologia* 3, no. 2 (1967): 238–48.

52. T. Coleman, "Obituary of Douglas L. Coleman 1931–2014," *Diabetologia* 57, no. 12 (2014): 2429–30.

4. THE ROCKEFELLER UNIVERSITY AND THE BROAD HORIZON

Note to Epigraph: Sir John Bell is the Regius Professor of Medicine at the University of Oxford.

1. E. L. Doctorow, "Afterword," in S. Lewis, *Arrowsmith* (New York: Signet Classics, 2008), 456. Paul de Kruif contributed much of the scientific language and culture to the text.

2. Lewis, *Arrowsmith*, 278.

3. Interview with David Luskutoff, March 2018.

4. Interview with Miki Rifkin, March 2018.

5. A. Cerami, "A Surprising Journey in Translational Medicine," *Molecular Medicine* 20 (2014): S3.

6. Cerami.

7. In 1977, American biochemist Eugene Goldwasser, at the University of Chicago, successfully isolated enough of the protein to allow the microsequencing of the amino terminus with newly discovered microsequencing technology.

8. C. Peterson and A. Cerami, "'Orphan-Drug' Development—Whose Responsibility?" *New England Journal of Medicine* 292, no. 3 (January 1975): 162.

9. Interview with Anthony Cerami, June 2018.

10. As early as the 1960s, it was acknowledged that inherited blood disorders of hemoglobin occur widely throughout the tropical world. Moreover, the relative neglect of the disease still continues. In 2010, Cerami's friend, British hematologist and thalassemia specialist Sir David Weatherall, wrote, "This problem is exacerbated by the fact that the WHO, other nongovernmental organizations and the major international charities have, with a few exceptions, shown no interest in genetic disease, focusing almost entirely on the major communicable diseases." D. Weatherall, "Thalassemia: The Long Road from the Bedside through the Laboratory to the Community," *Nature Medicine* 16, no. 10 (October 2010): xxvi.

11. D. Weatherall, ed., *Advanced Medicine* 14 (London: Pitman Medical, 1978), 332.

12. Interview with Joseph Graziano, October 2017.

13. D. Bergsma, A. Cerami, C. Peterson, and J. Graziano, eds., *Iron Metabolism and Thalassemia. Birth Defects: Original Article Series* 12, no. 8 (New York: Alan R. Liss, 1976).

14. C. Peterson, J. Graziano, R. Grady, R. Jones, H. Vlassara, V. Canale, D. Miller, and A. Cerami, "Chelation Studies with 2,3-Dihydroxybenzoic Acid in Patients with β-Thalassemia Major," *British Journal of Haematology* 33, no. 4 (1976): 477–85.

15. Interview with Joseph Graziano, October 2017.

16. A. Cerami, "The Value of Failure: The Discovery of TNF and Its Natural Inhibitor Erythropoietin," *Journal of Internal Medicine* 269, no. 1 (2011): 8–15.

17. Interview with Daniel Rifkin, October 2017.

18. Interview with Joseph Graziano, October 2017.

19. J. Graziano and E. Friedheim, "The Pharmacology of 2,3-Dimercaptosuccinic Acid (DMS): A New Agent for the Treatment of Heavy Metal Poisoning," *Paediatric Research* 12, no. 406 (1978): 254.

20. P. Flint, "Ernst Friedheim, 89, Developer of Drugs for Ills of the Tropics," *New York Times*, May 31, 1989.

21. Interview with Joseph Graziano, October 2017.

22. C. Moberg, *Rene Dubos, Friend of the Good Earth: Microbiologist, Medical Scientist, Environmentalist* (Washington, D.C.: ASM Press, 2005), 69.

23. P. de Kruif, *Microbe Hunters* (New York: Harcourt, Brace and Company, 1926), 234.

24. E. West, "Things Come Together: Science and the American West," Harmsworth Lecture, University of Oxford (November 7, 2017).

25. Interview with Elliott West, November 2017.

26. de Kruif, *Microbe Hunters*, 250.

27. Interview with Anthony Cerami, June 2018.

28. C. Spence, *Gastrophysics: The New Science of Eating* (London: Viking, 2017).

29. Interview with Anthony Cerami, June 2016.

30. Interview with Barbara Luskutoff, March 2018.

31. P. Medawar, "Lucky Jim" [review of J. Watson, *The Double Helix*], *New York Review of Books*, March 28, 1968. See also P. Medawar, "Is the Scientific Paper a Fraud?" *Listener* 70 (1963): 377–78.

32. Interview with Anthony Cerami, June 2018.

33. Interview with John Bell, April 2016.

5. DIABETES

1. A. Cerami, "The Value of Failure: The Discovery of TNF and Its Natural Inhibitor Erythropoietin," *Journal of Internal Medicine* 269, no. 1 (2011): 8–15.

2. A. Cerami, "The Unexpected Pathway to the Creation of the HbA1c Test and the Discovery of AGEs," *Journal of Internal Medicine* 271, no. 3 (2012): 219–21.

3. R. Nalbandian, R. Henry, B. Nichols, D. Kessler, F. Camp Jr., and K. Vining, "The Molecular Basis for the Treatment of Sickle Cell Crisis by Intravenous Urea," *Annals of Internal Medicine* 72 (1970): 795.

4. There is only one amino acid difference between sickle cell hemoglobin and normal hemoglobin involving the substitution of a negatively charged amino acid with a hydrophobic amino acid. When the oxygen is given up by the hemoglobin molecule, it changes its confirmation and will react with other hydrophobic elements and forms polymers that cause the cells to sickle.

5. Interview with Carol Rouser, May 2017.

6. Interview with Anthony Cerami, June 2018.

7. G. Stark, W, Stein, and S. Moore, "Reactions of the Cyanate Present in Aqueous Urea with Amino Acids and Proteins," *Journal of Biological Chemistry* 235 (1960): 3177–81.

8. A. Cerami and J. Manning, "Potassium Cyanate as an Inhibitor of the Sickling of Erythrocytes in vitro," *Proceedings of the National Academy of Sciences of the United States of America* 68, no. 6 (1971): 1180–83.

9. P. Gillette, J. Manning, and A. Cerami, "Increased Survival of Sickle-Cell Erythrocytes after Treatment In Vitro with Sodium Cyanate," *Proceedings of the National Academy of Sciences of the United States of America* 68, no. 11 (1971): 2791–93.

10. Interview with Charles Dinarello, February 2017.

11. Interview with David Weatherall, April 2016.

12. Interview with Anthony Cerami, June 2016.

13. P. Gillette, C. Peterson, Y. Lu, and A. Cerami, "Sodium Cyanate as a Potential Treatment for Sickle-Cell Disease," *New England Journal of Medicine* 290, no. 12 (1974): 654–60.

14. Interview with David Weatherall, May 2017.

15. A. Cerami, "A Surprising Journey in Translational Medicine," *Molecular Medicine* 20 (2014): S2–S6.

16. A. Flexner, *The Usefulness of Useless Knowledge (with a Companion Essay by Robbert Dijkgraaf)* (Princeton, NJ: Princeton University Press, 2017), 57.

17. S. Rahbar, "An Abnormal Haemoglobin in Red Cells of Diabetes," *Clinica Chimica Acta* 22, no. 2 (1968): 296–98.

18. L. Trivelli, H. Ranney, and H. Lai, "Hemoglobin Components in Patients with Diabetes Mellitus," *New England Journal of Medicine* 284, no. 7 (1971): 353–57.

19. Interview with Anthony Cerami, June 2018.

20. Interview with Anthony Cerami, June 2018.

21. Interview with Ronald Koenig, May 2017.

22. Interview with Ronald Koenig, May 2017.

23. Interview with Kirk Manogue, May 2016.

24. Interview with Anthony Cerami, June 2018.

25. Interview with Anthony Cerami, June 2018.

26. Cerami, "Unexpected Pathway," 219–26.

27. Interview with Ronald Koenig, May 2017.

28. Interview with Ronald Koenig, May 2017.

29. Interview with James Gowans, December 2013.

30. Interview with Ronald Koenig, May 2017.

31. R. Koenig and A. Cerami, "Synthesis of Hemoglobin AIc in Normal and Diabetic Mice: Potential Model of Basement Membrane Thickening," *Proceedings of the National Academy of Sciences of the United States of America* 72, no. 9 (1975): 3687–91.

32. Interview with Ronald Koenig, May 2017.

33. R. Koenig, S. Blobstein, and A. Cerami, "Structure of Carbohydrate of Hemoglobin AIc," *Journal of Biological Chemistry* 252, no. 9 (1977): 2992–97.

34. The structure of hemoglobin A1c is the same as that as hemoglobin A except for the addition of a carbohydrate moiety as the amino terminal valine of the beta chain.

35. Interview with Gerald Bernstein, June 2016.

36. Interview with Ronald Koenig, May 2017.

37. For much of the second half of the twentieth century, the question of hyperglycemia divided medical opinion in the United States—were complications independent of, or a consequence of, diabetic hyperglycemia? In the "independent" corner was Dr. Edward Tolstoi, who believed that hyperglycemia was not relevant to the patient's health, and one should not worry unduly about blood glucose level. For the "consequence" view was Dr. Elliott P. Joslin, who advocated that the tight control of hyperglycemia would delay or prevent complications. "Food," said Dr. Joslin, "is a medicine like insulin, and must be precisely prescribed and measured."

38. Cerami, "Unexpected Pathway," 220.

39. Interview with Ronald Koenig, May 2017.

40. R. Koenig, C. Peterson, R. Jones, C. Saudek, M. Lehrman, and A. Cerami, "Correlation of Glucose Regulation and Hemoglobin A1c in Diabetes Mellitus," *New England Journal of Medicine* 295, no. 8 (1976): 417–20.

41. Interview with Anthony Cerami, June 2018.

42. Interview with David Weatherall, April 2016.

43. Interview with Anthony Cerami, June 2018.

44. Interview with Anthony Cerami, June 2018.

45. Interview with Charles Dinarello, February 2017.

46. L. Jovanovic and C. Peterson, "Management of the Pregnant, Insulin-Dependent Diabetic Woman," *Diabetes Care* 3, no. 1 (1980): 63–68.

47. The Diabetes Control and Complications Trial Research Group, "The Effect of Intensive Treatment of Diabetes on the Development and Progression of Long-term Complications in Insulin-dependent Diabetes Mellitus," *New England Journal of Medicine* 329 (1993): 977–86.

48. UK Prospective Diabetes Study Group, "Tight Blood Pressure Control and Risk of Macrovascular and Microvascular Complications in Type 2 Diabetes: UKPDS 38," *British Medical Journal* 317 (1998): 703–13.

49. M. Brownlee, H. Vlassara, A. Kooney, P. Ulrich, and A. Cerami, "Aminoguanidine Prevents Diabetes-Induced Arterial Wall Protein Cross-linking," *Science* 232, no. 4758 (1986): 1629–32.

50. Interview with Charles Dinarello, February 2017.

6. GLUCOSE, AGING, AND THE CROSS-LINKING OF BIOLOGY AND BUSINESS

1. P. Medawar, *The Art of the Soluble: Creativity and Originality in Science* (London: Methuen, 1967).

2. A. Cerami, "Advances in Medical Science," in *On the Brink of Tomorrow: Frontiers of Science*, ed. D. de Solla (Washington, D.C.: National Geographic Society, 1982), 148.

3. Interview with Joseph Graziano, October 2017.

4. H. Vlassara, M. Brownlee, and A. Cerami, "Nonenzymatic Glycosylation and the Pathogenesis of Diabetic Complications," *Annals of Internal Medicine* 101, no. 4 (1984): 527.

5. A. Cerami, "Hypothesis. Glucose as a Mediator of Aging," *Journal of the American Geriatrics Society* 33, no. 9 (1985): 632.

6. Cerami, "Advances in Medical Science," 148.

7. R. Doll and R. Peto, "There Is No Such Thing as Aging: Old Age Is Associated with Disease, but Does Not Cause It," *British Medical Journal* 315, no. 7115 (1997): 1030–32.

8. Doll and Peto, 1030.

9. L. Vikhanski, *Immunity: How Elie Metchnikoff Changed the Course of Modern History* (Chicago: Chicago Review Press, 2016), 259.

10. J. Cairns, *Matters of Life and Death: Perspectives on Public Health, Molecular Biology, Cancer, and the Prospects for the Human Race* (Princeton, NJ: Princeton University Press, 1997), 3.

11. C. Keating, "The Genesis of the Global Burden of Disease Study," *Lancet* 391, no. 10137 (2018): 2316–17.

12. Vikhanski, *Immunity*, 154.

13. Vikhanski, 264.

14. S. Vasan, X. Zhang, X. Zhang, et al., "An Agent Cleaving Glucose-Derived Protein Crosslinks In Vitro and In Vivo," *Nature* 382, no. 6588 (1996): 275–78.

15. B. Ehrenreich, *Living with a Wild God: A Nonbeliever's Search for the Truth about Everything* (London: Granta Books, 2014), 170.

16. V. Stevens, C. Rouzer, V. Monnier, and A. Cerami, "Diabetic Cataract Formation: Potential Role of Glycosylation of Lens Crystallins," *Proceedings of the National Academy of Sciences of the United States of America* 75, no. 6 (1978): 2918–22.

17. Interview with Carol Rouzer, May 2017.

18. A. Cerami, "The Unexpected Pathway to the Creation of the HbA1c Test and the Discovery of AGEs," *Journal of Internal Medicine* 271, no. 3 (2012): 219–26.

19. Interview with Carol Rouser, May 2017.

20. Interview with Anthony Cerami, June 2018.

21. Interview with Carol Rouser, May 2017.

22. Interview with Carol Rouser, May 2017.

23. Interview with Vincent Monnier, October 2017.

24. Interview with Vincent Monnier, October 2017.

25. V. Stevens, V. Monnier, and A. Cerami, "Hemoglobin Glycosylation as a Model for Modification of Other Proteins," *Texas Reports on Biology and Medicine* 40 (1980): 387–96.

26. Jo Thomasung, *New York Times*, August 13, 1979.

27. C. Cerami, H. Founds, I. Nicholl, et al., "Tobacco Smoke Is a Source of Toxic Reactive Glycation Products," *Proceedings of the National Academy of Sciences of the United States of America* 94, no. 25 (1997): 13915–20.

28. H. Vlassara and S. Woodruff, *The A.G.E. Food Guide: A Quick Reference to Foods and the A.G.E.s They Contain* (New York: SquareOne Publishers, 2017), 14.

29. Interview with Vincent Monnier, October 2017.

30. Vlassara and Woodruff, *The A.G.E. Food Guide*, 16.

31. H. Vlassara, J. Uribarri, G. Striker, and S. Woodruff, *The AGE-Less Way: Escape America's Over-Eating Epidemic* (Lexington, KY: Createspace, 2012).

32. Vlassara and Woodruff, *The A.G.E. Food Guide*, 15.

33. Interview with Carla Cerami, May 2018.

34. Interview with Carla Cerami, May 2018.

35. Interview with Vincent Monnier, October 2017.

36. Interview with Joseph Graziano, October 2018.

37. Interview with Alan Fairlamb, May 2016.

38. Interview with Miki Rifkin, March 2018.

39. Interview with Vincent Monnier, October 2017.

40. Interview with Anthony Cerami, June 2018.

41. Cerami, "Hypothesis," 626–34.

42. "Obituary: Robert Butler," *British Medical Journal* 341 (2010): c4051.

43. "Obituary: Robert Butler," *The Guardian*, July 18, 2010.

44. Interview with Michael Brownlee, October 2017.

45. Stanford Moore shared the Nobel Prize in 1972 with Christian Anfinsen and William H. Stein for work done at Rockefeller University. In 1959, Moore and Stein announced the first determination of the complete amino acid sequence of an enzyme, ribonuclease, and the development of chromatography.

46. R. Severo, "Stanford Moore, a Nobel Laureate," *New York Times*, August 24, 1982.

47. Cerami, "Unexpected Pathway," 225.

48. G. Owens and T. Hollis, "Relationship between Inhibition of Aortic Histamine Formation, Aortic Albumin Permeability and Atherosclerosis," *Atherosclerosis* 34, no. 4 (1979): 365–73.

49. Interview with Michael Brownlee, October 2017.

50. Cerami, "Unexpected Pathway," 225.

51. M. Brownlee, H. Vlassara, A. Kooney, P. Ulrich, and A. Cerami, "Aminoguanidine Prevents Diabetes-Induced Arterial Wall Protein Cross-linking," *Science* 232, no. 4758 (1986): 1629–32.

52. H. Schmeck Jr., "Experimental Drug Raises Hope on Diabetes," *New York Times*, July 20, 1986.

53. Brownlee et al., "Aminoguanidine," 1632.

54. A. Cerami, "A Surprising Journey in Translational Medicine," *Molecular Medicine* 20 (2014): S4.

55. G. Ferry, "Obituary of Sir John Sulston," *The Guardian*, March 12, 2018.

56. Interview with Anthony Cerami, December 2018.

57. Although all medical research is by nature incremental, occasionally a discovery is made that causes profound and immediate change. Just such a moment occurred in 1975, when Georges Kohler and Cesar Milstein, scientists working at the University of Cambridge, published a three-page article in *Nature* and announced the discovery of monoclonal antibodies. The article concluded with a prophetic sentence: "Such cultures could be valuable for medical and industrial use." The later debates and recriminations about the apparent failure of British science and technology to exploit this invention to commercial advantage threw monoclonal antibodies into a public prominence rarely achieved by scientific discoveries. The sense of failure to get a patent for Kohler and Milstein's hybridoma technique, which would have provided much-needed funds for British biomedical research, turned to anger with the granting of two patents to Hilary Koprowski, Carlo Croce, and Walter Gerhard at the Wistar Institute in Philadelphia for the making of monoclonal antibodies against tumors and influenza virus in October 1979 and April 1980. These were the world's first patents awarded for the making of a monoclonal antibody. The patents were subsequently licensed to U.S. biotechnology company Centocor, in which the Wistar scientists held significant parts of the shares.

58. S. Schweitzer, *Pharmaceutical Economics and Policy* (New York: Oxford University Press, 2007), 59.

59. A. Cerami, H. Vlassara, and M. Brownlee, "Glucose and Aging," *Scientific American* 256, no. 5 (1987): 90–96.

60. Schweitzer, *Pharmaceutical Economics*, 59.

61. H. Harris, "Florey and Penicillin," *Oxford Magazine* 158 (1998): 1–5.

62. Interview with Richard Bucala, August 2018.

63. Interview with Vincent Monnier, October 2017.

64. C. Keating, "Introducing a History of Key Trials in *The Lancet*," *Lancet* 390, no. 10107 (2017): 2025.

65. W. Bolton, D. Cattran, M. Williams, et al., "Randomized Trial of an Inhibitor of Formation of Advanced Glycation End Products in Diabetic Nephropathy," *American Journal of Nephrology* 24, no. 1 (2004): 32–40.

66. The great and the good from Fisher to Neyman and Kolmogorov would argue what a significance test is and what probability means. Usually in a trial of two treatments, for example, say you have stated a prior null hypothesis that is to be tested—typically, it is that the treatments have the same effect on some specified disease. The effect can be measured as a rate (e.g., disease rate per year) or a risk (X out of N individuals got the disease). So the null hypothesis would be that at the end of the study, the disease rates (or risks) are the same in both treatment groups. The significance test is a (indirect) measure of the degree to which the data in your trial contradict your null hypothesis that the disease rates in the two treatments arms are the same. The smaller the p-value, the greater the contradiction. If the study is small, you may just get a small p-value due to chance.

67. Cerami, "Unexpected Pathway," 225.

68. Bolton et al., "Randomized Trial," 32–40.

69. Interview with Anthony Cerami, June 2018.

70. Cerami, "Unexpected Pathway," 225.

71. Cerami, "Surprising Journey," S2–S6.

72. Interview with Anthony Cerami, June 2018.

73. Interview with Anthony Cerami, December 2018.

74. K. Tracey, "Molecular Medicine Commemorates the Career and Science of Anthony Cerami," *Molecular Medicine* 20 (2014): S1.

7. THE CONCEPTUAL BREAKTHROUGH

1. In a letter dated July 13, 1976, to British parasitologist George Cross of the Molteno Institute, University of Cambridge, Cerami wrote, "Bill Trager told me of your upcoming visit to New York and I am pleased that we will be able to host you during your stay at The Rockefeller University. . . . I mentioned to C. C. Wang of the Merck Institute of Therapeutics about your upcoming visit to the United States and he asked if it would be possible for you to schedule a day when you could visit his laboratory in New Jersey. They have recently embarked on a program to study Trypanosomiasis and would like very much to talk with you." A little over a year later (July 20, 1977), Cerami, who would subsequently recruit Cross to the faculty of The Rockefeller University, wrote, "I recently heard from John Ryley that you are planning to leave the Molteno Institute to go with Wellcome. I hope that this does not mean that you will be abandoning the field of parasitology in this move. You are doing some of the most interesting work in the field and we would hate to see you desert us."

2. G. Nossal, "Book Review: C. Keating, *Kenneth Warren and the Great Neglected Diseases of Mankind Programme: The Transformation of Geographical Medicine in the US and Beyond*," *International Journal of Epidemiology* 46, no. 6 (2017): 2100–2.

3. G. Mitchell, "Comments on the GND Program" in *The Great Neglected Diseases of Mankind Biomedical Research Network: 1978–1988*, ed. K. Warren and C. Jimenez (New York: The Rockefeller Foundation, 1988), 49.

4. C. Keating, *Kenneth Warren and the Great Neglected Diseases of Mankind Programme: The Transformation of Geographical Medicine in the US and Beyond* (Cham, Switzerland: Springer, 2017), xvi.

5. R. Zelzer, "Obituary of Kenneth S. Warren," *Molecular Medicine* 2, no. 6 (1996).

6. D. Weatherall, "Introduction," in Keating, *Kenneth Warren*, v.

7. Warren and Jimenez, *Great Neglected Diseases*, 1.

8. Nossal, "Book Review."

9. Warren and Jimenez, *Great Neglected Diseases*, 1.

10. K. Warren, "The Bench and the Bush in Tropical Medicine," *American Journal of Tropical Medicine and Hygiene* 30, no. 6 (1981): 1149–58.

11. Warren and Jimenez, *Great Neglected Diseases*, 119.

12. Warren and Jimenez, 119.

13. Interview with John Bell, April 2016.

14. L. Miller, "The Impact of Ken Warren's Leadership of the Rockefeller Foundation's Great Neglected Diseases Program on the Future of Malaria Research," *American Journal of Tropical Medicine and Hygiene* 97, no. 6 (2017): 1958.

15. Weatherall, "Introduction," v.

16. Warren and Jimenez, *Great Neglected Diseases*, 120.

17. Warren and Jimenez, 2.

18. Some of the outstanding scientists from the global south who contributed to the GND science included Ulisses Lopes, a scientist in Rio de Janeiro, Brazil, working on *Leishmania* who earned a PhD at the Harvard School of Public Health; Anastaçio Sousa and Jose Wellingon Lima from Ceará, Brazil; Mitermayer des Mitermayer des Reis, head of FIOCRUZ in Salvador and expert on schistosomiasis; and Carlos Morel, president of FIOCRUZ and Chair Committee of WHO/TDR for funding new centers.

19. Interview with Steve Meshnick, April 2015.

20. Anthony Cerami's acceptance speech for the award of the Paul Ehrlich Prize in Frankfurt (March 14, 2018).

21. S. Meshnick, S. Blobstein, R. Grady, and A. Cerami, "An Approach to the Development of New Drugs for African Trypanosomiasis," *Journal of Experimental Medicine* 148, no. 2 (1978): 567–79.

22. A. Fairlamb, P. Blackburn, P. Ulrich, B. Chait, and A. Cerami, "Trypanothione: A Novel Bis(glutathionyl) Spermidine Cofactor for Glutathione Reductase in Trypanosomatids," *Science* 227, no. 4693 (1985): 1485–87.

23. Interview with Steve Meshnick, April 2015.

24. A. Cerami, "A Forty-Year Odyssey in the Sea of Translational Medicine," *Proceedings of the American Philosophical Society* 158, no. 4 (December 2014): 404.

25. S. Blobstein, R. Grady, S. Meshnick, and A. Cerami, "Hydroxamic Acid Oxidation—Pharmacological Considerations," *Biochemical Pharmacology* 27, no. 24 (1978): 2939–45.

26. Interview with Anthony Cerami, June 2018.

27. Cerami, "Forty-Year Odyssey."

28. P. Medawar, *Advice to a Young Scientist* (New York: Harper & Row, 1979).

29. For a written record of the meeting, see K. Warren and J. Bowers, eds., *Parasitology: A Global Perspective: Proceedings of a Meeting in Bellagio, Italy, April 1982* (New York: Springer, 1983).

30. The course, established in 1980, was the brainchild of Ken Warren, Joshua Lederberg, Joe Cook of the Edna McConnell Clark Foundation, and Cerami. The idea was to bring sixteen students from around the world, with special emphasis on students from the tropical belt, and to train them with the new tools and techniques that would bring a better understanding of their countries' indigenous diseases. The ten-week course attracted students who went on to celebrated careers in parasitology, including Dyann Wirth, Onesmo ole-MoiYoi, Norma Andrews, Photini Sine, and Ricardo Gazzinelli.

31. Detlev Bronk's speech in support of Cerami's candidacy for doctorate in philosophy.

32. L. Thomas, "Natural Science," in *The Lives of a Cell: Notes of a Biology Watcher* (New York: Viking, 1974), 100–103.

33. S. Meshnick, K. Chang, and A. Cerami, "Heme Lysis of the Bloodstream Forms of *Trypanosoma brucei*," *Biochemical Pharmacology* 26, no. 20 (1977): 1923–28.

34. L. Chang, E. Cheriathundam, E. Mahoney, and A. Cerami, "DNA Polymerases in Parasitic Protozoans Differ from Host Enzymes," *Science* 208, no. 4443 (1980): 510–11.

35. Warren and Jimenez, *Great Neglected Diseases*, 197.

36. Interview with Steve Meshnick, April 2015.

37. A. Cerami, "The Value of Failure: The Discovery of TNF and Its Natural Inhibitor Erythropoietin," *Journal of Internal Medicine* 269, no. 1 (2011): 9.

38. Cerami, "Value of Failure," 8.

39. Interview with Anthony Cerami, June 2018.

40. Interview with Anthony Cerami, June 2018.

41. Interview with Anthony Cerami, June 2018.

42. Interview with Steve Meshnick, April 2015.

43. Cerami, "Value of Failure," 10.

44. From the poem "Stufen" (Steps) written by Hermann Hesse in 1941.

45. C. Panosian and P. Rosenthal, "'The Way We Were': Ken Warren's Legacy and Modern Investments in Global Health," American Journal of Tropical Medicine and Hygiene 97, no. 6 (2017): 1955–57.

46. F. Crick, What Mad Pursuit: A Personal View of Scientific Discovery (London: Weidenfeld and Nicholson, 1989). The title is from a line in the poem "Ode of a Grecian Urn" by John Keats. The book's title is from line 9 of the poem—intriguingly, line 10 contains the phrase "What struggle to escape."

47. Interview with Alan Fairlamb, May 2016.

48. Interview with Carol Rouser, May 2017.

49. Cerami, "Value of Failure," 8.

50. Interview with Carol Rouser, May 2017.

51. C. Rouser and A. Cerami, "Hypertriglyceridemia Associated with Trypanosoma brucei brucei Infection in Rabbits: Role of Defective Triglyceride Removal," Molecular and Biological Parasitology 2, no. 1 (1980): 31–38.

52. E. Mahoney, A. Hamil, W. Scott, and Z. Cohn, "Response of Endocytosis to Altered Fatty Acyl Composition of Macrophage Phospholipids," Proceedings of the National Academy of Sciences of the United States of America 74, no. 11 (1977): 4895–99.

53. Interview with Anthony Cerami, June 2018.

54. Interview with Alan Fairlamb, May 2016.

55. Interview with Keith McAdam, October 2016.

56. Interview with Carol Rouser, May 2017.

57. Cerami, "Value of Failure," 8–15.

58. V. Lobo, A. Patel, A. Phatak, and N. Chandra, "Free Radicals, Antioxidants and Functional Foods: Impact on Human Health," Pharmacognosy Reviews 4, no. 8 (2010): 118–26.

59. Interview with Carol Rouser, May 2017.

60. Interview with Alan Fairlamb, May 2016.

61. Cerami, "Value of Failure," 9.

62. Interview with Masanobu Kawakami, August 2017.

63. M. Kawakami, "Discovery of Tumor Necrosis Factor (TNF) and Identification of the Potential of Anti-TNF Antibodies in Dr. Cerami's Laboratory," Molecular Medicine 20 (2014): S18.

64. B. Sultzer, "Genetic Control of Leucocyte Responses to Endotoxin," Nature 219, no. 5160 (1968): 1253.

65. Cerami, "Value of Failure," 10.

66. Kawakami, "Discovery of Tumor Necrosis Factor," S18.

67. Interviw with Masanobu Kawakami, August 2017.

68. Z. Cohn, "The Regulation of Pinocytosis in Mouse Macrophages: I. Metabolic Requirements as Defined by the Use of Inhibitors," Journal of Experimental Medicine 124, no. 4 (1966): 557–71.

69. C. Moberg, Entering an Unseen World: A Founding Laboratory and Origins of Modern Cell Biology, 1910–1974 (New York: The Rockefeller University Press, 2012), 327.

70. Kawakami, "Discovery of Tumor Necrosis Factor," S18.

71. M. Kawakami, P. Pekala, M. Lane, and A. Cerami, "Selective Inhibition of Synthesis of Enzymes for De Novo Fatty Acid Biosynthesis by an Endotoxin-Induced Mediator from Exudate Cells," Proceedings of the National Academy of Sciences of the United States of America 80, no. 9 (1983): 2743–47.

72. S. Sassa, M. Kawakami, and A. Cerami, "Inhibition of the Growth and Differentiation of Erythroid Precursor Cells by an Endotoxin-Induced Mediator from Peritoneal Macrophages," *Proceedings of the National Academy of Sciences of the United States of America* 80, no. 6 (1983): 1717–20.

73. Kawakami, "Discovery of Tumor Necrosis Factor," S18.

74. L. O'Neill, *Humanology: A Scientist's Guide to Our Amazing Existence* (Dublin: Gill Books, 2018), 251.

75. Interview with Anthony Cerami, June 2018.

76. Interview with Anthony Cerami, June 2018.

77. Interview with Masanobu Kawakami, August 2017.

78. A. Cerami, "A Surprising Journey in Translational Medicine," *Molecular Medicine* 20 (2014): S4.

79. Interview with Anthony Cerami, June 2018.

80. Interview with Masanobu Kawakami, August 2017. M. Kawakami and A. Cerami, "Studies of Endotoxin-Induced Decrease in Lipoprotein Lipase Activity," *Journal of Experimental Medicine* 154, no. 3 (1981): 631–39.

81. A. Cerami and M. Kawakami, "Method for Reducing Adverse Effects of a Human 70kDa Mediator Which Results from Endotoxin Stimulation of Macrophages," U.S. Patent # 6419927 BI.

82. Interview with Charles Dinarello, February 2017.

8. CACHECTIN-TUMOR NECROSIS FACTOR

1. J. Cairns, *Matters of Life and Death: Perspectives on Public Health, Molecular Biology, Cancer, and the Prospects for the Human Race* (Princeton, NJ: Princeton University Press, 1997), 3.

2. F. Breedveld, "TNF Antagonists Opened the Way to Personalized Medicine in Rheumatoid Arthritis," *Molecular Medicine* 20 (2014): S9.

3. Letter from Cerami to Joshua Lederberg, March 5, 1985 (Anthony Cerami personal papers).

4. On August 24, 1982, Tony Cerami wrote to his colleague, Dr. Attallah Kappas, professor and physician-in-chief at the Rockefeller Hospital: "I recently had several meetings with Ernie Beutler of Scripps, and wondered whether the Clinical Committee might consider his candidacy for a position in the Hospital. As I am sure you are aware, Ernie has been one of the outstanding haematologists in the world and continues to have an active research program, which is exemplary for the application of modern science to medical problems. If you thought that it would be of interest, I would [be] pleased to obtain his C.V. for your consideration. I am not sure how moveable Ernie is at the present time, but I do know that most of his funding at Scripps, including his salary, is derived from grant support. He might be wanting to change that type of arrangement. I look forward to hearing from you."

5. Letter from Cerami to Masanobu Kawakami, August 24, 1982 (Anthony Cerami personal papers).

6. Letter from Bruce Beutler to Cerami, August 17, 1982 (Anthony Cerami personal papers).

7. G. Fantuzzi, *Body Messages: The Quest for the Proteins of Cellular Communication* (Cambridge, MA: Harvard University Press, 2016), 78.

8. Letter from Cerami to Joshua Lederberg, March 5, 1985 (Anthony Cerami personal papers).

9. B. Beutler, J. Mahoney, N. Le Trang, P. Pekala, and A. Cerami, "Purification of Cachectin, a Lipoprotein Lipase-Suppressing Hormone Secreted by Endotoxin-Induced RAW 264.7 Cells," *Journal of Experimental Medicine* 161, no. 5 (1985): 984–95.

10. B. Aggarwal, W. Kohr, E. Hass, et al., "Human Necrosis Factor: Production, Purification and Characterization," *Journal of Biological Chemistry* 260 (1985): 2345–54.

11. Fantuzzi, *Body Messages*, 79.

12. C. Keating, *Smoking Kills: The Revolutionary Life of Richard Doll* (Oxford: Signal Books, 2009), 89.

13. E. Carswell, L. Old, R. Kassel, S. Green, N. Fiore, and B. Williamson, "An Endotoxin-Induced Serum Factor That Causes Necrosis of Tumors," *Proceedings of the National Academy of Sciences of the United States of America* 72, no. 9 (1975): 3666–70.

14. M. Kawakami, "Discovery of Tumor Necrosis Factor (TNF) and Identification of the Potential of Anti-TNF Antibodies in Dr. Cerami's Laboratory," *Molecular Medicine* 20 (2014): S19.

15. Interview with Anthony Cerami, June 2018.

16. M. Smyth, "Lloyd John Old 1933–2011," *Nature Immunology* 13 (2012): 103.

17. W. Coley, "The Treatment of Malignant Tumors by Repeated Inoculations of Erysipelas: With Report of Ten Original Cases," *American Journal of the Medical Sciences* 105 (1893): 487–94.

18. Fantuzzi, *Body Messages*, 79.

19. Interview with Barbara Sherry, May 2016.

20. B. Beutler and A. Cerami, "Cachectin and Tumor Necrosis Factor as Two Sides of the Same Coin," *Nature* 320 (1980): 584–88.

21. Beutler and Cerami, 587.

22. A. Cerami and B. Beutler, "Cachectin: The Dark Side of Tumor Necrosis Factor," in *Molecular Biology of Homo Sapiens: Cold Spring Harbor Symposium on Quantitative Biology*, vol. 51 (New York: Cold Spring Harbor Press, 1986), 625–29.

23. H. Schmeck Jr., "Anticancer Substance Reveals its Dark Side," *New York Times*, December 9, 1986.

24. National Program for the Conquest of Cancer, *Report of the National Panel of Consultants on the Conquest of Cancer* (Washington, D.C.: Government Printing Office, 1970).

25. Keating, *Smoking Kills*, 339.

26. Interview with Anthony Cerami, June 2018.

27. Letter from Beutler and Cerami to Samuel Ackerman, June 19, 1985 (Anthony Cerami personal papers).

28. Letter from Beutler and Cerami to Karl Pinsly, June 15, 1985 (Anthony Cerami personal papers).

29. K. Tracey, *Fatal Sequence: The Killer Within* (New York: Dana Press, 2005).

30. Fantuzzi, *Body Messages*, 83.

31. B. Beutler, I. Milsark, and A. Cerami, "Passive Immunization against Cachectin/Tumor Necrosis Factor (TNF) Protects Mice from the Lethal Effect of Endotoxin," *Science* 229 (1985): 869–71.

32. Fantuzzi, *Body Messages*, 79.

33. Beutler et al., "Passive Immunization," 869.

34. Tracey, *Fatal Sequence*, 130.

35. I. Oransky, "Obituary of G. Tom Shires," *Lancet* 371 (2008): 200.

36. Shires was a surgeon at Dallas's Parkland Memorial Hospital in 1963 when President John Kennedy was shot. Shires successfully operated on Texas Governor John Connally for wounds he suffered during the assassination. Two days later, he operated on Lee Harvey Oswald, unsuccessfully, after Oswald was brought to the same emergency room in an ambulance without paramedics or saline.

37. Fantuzzi, *Body Messages*, 2.

38. Interview with Kevin Tracey, August 2017.

39. Tracey, *Fatal Sequence*, 131.

40. Interview with Kevin Tracey, August 2017.

41. Interview with Kevin Tracey, August 2017.

42. K. Tracey, B. Beutler, S. Lowry, et al., "Shock and Tissue Injury Induced by Recombinant Human Cachectin," *Science* 234, no. 4775 (1986): 470–74.

43. Fantuzzi, *Body Messages*, 89.

44. Tracey, *Fatal Sequence*, 133.

45. J. Bell, "The Double Helix in Clinical Practice," *Nature* 421, no. 6921 (2003): 414–16.

46. T. Lewis, "Reflections upon Medical Education," *Lancet* 1 (1944): 619–21.

47. B. Beutler and A. Cerami, "Cachectin (Tumor Necrosis Factor) and Lymphotoxin as Primary Mediators of Tissue Catabolism, Inflammation, and Shock," in *Lymphokines and the Immune Response*, ed. S. Cohen (Boca Raton, FL: CRC Press, 1990), 200–207.

48. Tracey, *Fatal Sequence*, 135.

49. Tracey, 136.

50. The researchers chose to use fragments of the antibody with the hope that the smaller fragments would get into the tissues faster and give a larger window in time since the mouse experiments showed the inability of complete antibodies to be effective in preventing death if given at the time of endotoxin administration.

51. Tracey, *Fatal Sequence*, 137.

52. Tracey, 138.

53. K. Tracey, Y. Fong, D. Hesse, et al., "Anti-Cachectin/TNF Monoclonal Antibodies Prevent Septic Shock during Lethal Bacteraemia in Baboons," *Nature* 330, no. 6149 (1987): 662–64.

54. Tracey, Fong, Hesse, et al., 662.

55. Letter from Cerami to William J. Rutter, November 12, 1987 (Anthony Cerami personal papers).

56. Interview with Kevin Tracey, August 2017.

57. In 1972, Porter shared the Nobel Prize in Physiology or Medicine with Gerald M. Edelman for determining the chemical structure of an antibody.

58. K. Patel, "Michael Neuberger Obituary," *The Guardian*, December 21, 2013.

59. He shared the Nobel Prize with Bob Horvitz and John Sulston.

60. Cesar Milstein and George Kohler shared the Nobel Prize in Physiology or Medicine in 1984 (both of the LMB) with the Danish immunologist Niels Kaj Jerne "for theories concerning the specificity in development and control of the immune system and the discovery of the principle for production of monoclonal antibodies."

61. Interview with Nicholas Proudfoot, May 2018.

62. Tracey, *Fatal Sequence*, 140.

63. Fantuzzi, *Body Messages*, 83.

64. Tracey, *Fatal Sequence*, 140.

65. Interview with Charles Dinarello, February 2017.

66. J. Cohen and J. Carlet, "INTERSEPT: An International, Multicenter, Placebo-Controlled Trial of Monoclonal Antibody to Human Tumor Necrosis Factor–Alpha in Patients With Sepsis. International Sepsis Trial Study Group," *Critical Care Medicine* 24, no. 9 (1996): 1431–40.

67. E. Abraham, R. Wunderlink, H. Silverman, et al., "Efficacy and Safety of Monoclonal Antibody to Human Tumor Necrosis Factor in Patients with Sepsis Syndrome: A Randomized Controlled, Double-Blind Multicenter Clinical Trial. TNF-Alpha MAb Sepsis Study Group," *Journal of the American Medical Association* 273, no. 12 (1995): 934–41.

68. Interview with Charles Dinarello, February 2017.

69. Y. Fong, K. Tracey, L. Moldawer, et al., "Antibodies to Cachectin/Tumor Necrosis Factor Reduce Interleukin 1 Beta and Interleukin 6 Appearance during Lethal Bacteremia," *Journal of Experimental Medicine* 170, no. 5 (1989): 1627–33.

70. Interview with Yuman Fong, November 2018.

71. Interview with Charles Dinarello, February 2017.

72. Interview with Charles Dinarello, February 2017.

73. Interview with David Weatherall, August 2018.

74. Interview with Carla Cerami, May 2018.

75. Interview with Charles Dinarello, February 2017.

76. Interview with Miki Rifkin, March 2018.

77. D. Kwaitkowski, J. Cannon, K. Manogue, A. Cerami, C. Dinarello, and B. Greenwood, "Tumor Necrosis Factor Production in Falciparum Malaria and Its Association with Schizont Rupture," *Clinical and Experimental Immunology* 77, no. 3 (1989): 361–66.

78. J. Dayer, B. Beutler, and A. Cerami, "Cachectin/Tumor Necrosis Factor Stimulates Collagenase and Prostaglandin E2 Production by Human Synovial Cells and Dermal Fibroblasts," *Journal of Experimental Medicine* 162, no. 6 (1985): 2163–68.

79. Cairns, *Matters of Life and Death*, xi.

80. Interview with Charles Dinarello, February 2017.

81. C. Keating, *Great Medical Discoveries: An Oxford Story* (Oxford: The Bodleian Library, 2013), 41.

9. LEAVING THE ROCKEFELLER UNIVERSITY

1. J. Rogers Hollingsworth, "Institutionalizing Excellence in Biomedical Research: The Case of The Rockefeller University" in *Creating a Tradition of Biomedical Research: Contributions to the History of The Rockefeller University*, ed. D. H. Stapleton (New York: The Rockefeller University Press, 2004), 47.

2. The eponymous "Judy Lynn Farm" was named after Cerami's sister, Judith. The young Tony made the farm's sign, which he cut from a piece of wood using a buzz saw and nailed it to a tree outside the lane leading to their property.

3. Interview with Miki Rifkin, March 2018.

4. The famous Shelter Island Conference, which took place June 2–4, 1947, brought together many of the greatest theoretical physicists in the United States, including Robert Oppenheimer, Richard Feynman, Linus Pauling, and Hans Bethe, to discuss some of the most perplexing mysteries in physics. The meeting was held in the Ram's Head Inn, on Shelter Island, just off Long Island one hundred miles from New York City. The historic meeting was organized by, among others, Duncan MacInnes, a physicist at the Rockefeller Institute.

5. Interview with Ronald Koenig, May 2017.

6. Interview with Barbara Sherry, May 2016.

7. P. Hotez, "The Medical Biochemistry of Poverty and Neglect," *Molecular Medicine* 20 (2014): S31–S36.

8. Interview with George Cross, March 2018.

9. Interview with Miki Rifkin, March 2018.

10. A. Cerami, "Advances in Medical Science," in *On the Brink of Tomorrow: Frontiers of Science*, ed. D. de Solla (Washington, D.C.: National Geographic Society, 1982), 148–69.

11. N. Heatley, *Penicillin and Luck: Good Fortune in the Development of the 'Miracle Drug'* (RCJT Books, 2004), 1.

12. Interview with Yuman Fong, November 2018.

13. Interview with Yuman Fong, November 2018.

14. A. Fairlamb, P. Blackburn, P. Ulrich, B. Chait, and A. Cerami, "Trypanothione: A Novel Bis(glutathionyl) Spermidine Cofactor for Glutathione Reductase in Trypanosomatids," *Science* 227, no. 4693 (1985): 1485–87.

15. Interview with Alan Fairlamb, May 2016.

16. Interview with Alan Fairlamb, May 2016.

17. Interview with Miki Rifkin, March 2018.

18. Interview with Kevin Tracey, August 2017.

19. Interview with Carol Rouser, May 2017.

20. A. Cerami, "A Surprising Journey in Translational Medicine," *Molecular Medicine* 20 (2014): S2–S6.

21. Interview with Alan Fairlamb, May 2016.

22. G. Johas, *The Circuit Riders: Rockefeller Money and the Rise of Modern Science* (New York: Norton, 1989), 342.

23. Interview with Dan Rifkin, October 2017.

24. Interview with Tom Coleman, May 2016.

25. Interview with James Gowans, June 2014.

26. Interview with Richard Bucala, July 2018.

27. C. Keating, *Kenneth Warren and the Great Neglected Diseases of Mankind Programme: The Transformation of Geographical Medicine in the US and Beyond* (Cham, Switzerland: Springer, 2017), 138.

28. Interview with Barbara Sherry, May 2016.

29. Interview with Kevin Marsh, November 2017.

30. Interview with Richard Bucala, July 2018.

31. Hollingsworth, "Institutionalizing Excellence," 47.

32. D. Kevles, *The Baltimore Case: A Trial of Politics, Science, and Character* (New York: Norton, 1998), 196.

33. Hollingsworth, "Institutionalizing Excellence," 48.

34. Kevles, *Baltimore Case,* 9.

35. S. Hall, "David Baltimore's Final Days," *Science* 254, no. 5038 (1991): 1576.

36. Interview with Anthony Cerami, June 2016.

37. D. Weaver, M. Reis, C. Albanese, F. Costantini, D. Baltimore, and T. Imanishi-Kari, "Altered Repertoire of Endogenous Immunoglobulin Gene Expression in Transgenic Mice Containing a Rearranged Mu Heavy Chain Gene," *Cell* 45, no. 2 (1986): 247–59.

38. P. Hilts, "How Investigation of Lab Fraud Grew into a Cause Celebre," *New York Times,* March 26, 1991.

39. Kevles, *Baltimore Case.*

40. P. Doty, "Responsibility and Weaver et al," *Nature* 352, no. 6332 (1991): 183–84.

41. P. Elmer-DeWitt, "Thin Skins and Fraud at M. I. T.," *Time,* April 1, 1991, 65.

42. In the preface to his 1998 book *The Baltimore Case,* Daniel J. Kevles wrote, "Eventually, I became persuaded that Imanishi-Kari was innocent of the charges against her and said so in an article that appeared in *The New Yorker* magazine in May 1996. In subsequently writing this book, I found no reason to modify the fundamental judgements expressed there—except to have been reinforced in them by the outcome of the case. In June 1996, Thereza Imanishi-Kari was officially exonerated on all the counts that had been brought against her. David Baltimore began to re-enter public life, and in 1997 he was appointed president of the California Institute of Technology."

43. In June 1996, Thereza Imanishi-Kari was officially exonerated on all the counts that had been brought against her.

44. Kevles, *Baltimore Case,* 196.

45. Interview with Kirk Manogue, May 2016.

46. Elmer-DeWitt, "Thin Skins," 65.

47. Baltimore accepted the offer of the presidency on October 17, 1989. That day, in a speech to the faculty, he mentioned that in retrospect, he might have dealt with certain events differently, declaring, however, "I believe that by confronting Chairman Dingell directly, I was acting in the interests of all scientists. Only time will tell."

48. Hollingsworth, "Institutionalizing Excellence," 49.

49. M. Jacoby, "Foundations' Founder Yet to Donate $67-million," *St Petersburg Times,* December 29, 2001.

50. M. Jacoby, "Complex Web Benefits Foundation Founder," *St Petersburg Times,* July 8, 2001.

51. I. Edwards, "How a Major Research Institute Got to Long Island," *New York Times,* September 1, 1991.

52. Hall, "David Baltimore's Final Days," 1576.

53. In December 1991, following weeks of behind-the-scenes turmoil, president David Baltimore submitted his resignation to Rockefeller University's board of trustees—ending his

eighteenth-month term in office. "The reason I have decided to take this step," Baltimore said in his letter, "is that the *Cell* paper controversy created a climate of unhappiness among some in the university that could not be dispelled."

10. PHILANTHROPY GOES AWRY

1. J. Comroe Jr., and R. Dripps, "Scientific Basis for the Support of Biomedical Science," *Science* 192, no. 4235 (1976): 105–11.
2. L. Thomas, "The Planning of Science," in *The Lives of a Cell: Notes of a Biology Watcher* (New York: Penguin, 1978), 115.
3. R. Smith, "Comroe and Dripps Revisited," *British Medical Journal* 295, no. 6610 (1987): 1404–7.
4. I. Edwards, "How a Major Research Institute Got to Long Island," *New York Times*, September 1, 1991.
5. Interview with Kevin Tracey, August 2017.
6. Edwards, "How a Major Research Institute."
7. Interview with Barbara Sherry, May 2017.
8. Interview with Yousef Al-abed, May 2017.
9. Interview with Richard Bucala, November 2018.
10. Interview with Barbara Sherry, May 2017.
11. Robert Maxwell was a British-born press baron, described by newspaper editor Roy Greenslade as "a mercurial man with a monstrous ego." In 1988, Maxwell purchased the American publishing firm Macmillan for $2.6 billion and immediately looked for someone with a love of literature and knowledge of modern biomedical science to help run his new acquisition. Kenneth Warren, with his interests in knowledge transference and integration of scientific and medical publishing, made him an ideal candidate for the post. In 1991, Maxwell drowned under mysterious circumstances when his luxurious yacht *Lady Ghislane* was cruising off the Canary Islands.
12. Warren edited Lewis Thomas's final collection of essays *The Fragile Species* in 1992, which was published by Scribner.
13. Interview with Kevin Tracey, August 2017.
14. The journal was published in cooperation with Blackwell Scientific.
15. After the demise of the Picower Institute of Molecular Research, the graduate program was run by a new entity, the Elmezzi Graduate School of Molecular Medicine, an integral part of the Feinstein Institute and Northwell Health—now the largest health care system in New York State. One element of historical continuity is that the dean of the Elmezzi Graduate School today is Annette Lee.
16. M. Vitek, E. Stopa, F. Salles, et al., "Advanced Glycation End-Products Contribute to Amyloidosis in Alzheimer's Disease," in *Research Advances in Alzheimer's Disease and Related Disorders*, ed. K. Iqbal, J. Mortimer, B. Winblad, and H. Wisniewski (New York: John Wiley, 1995).
17. Cerami's team found high circulating levels of macrophage migration inhibitory factor in the blood of animals exposed to endotoxin. This material was produced in large quantities in the pituitary gland and macrophages. See also J. Bernhagen, T. Calandrea, R. Mitchell, A. Cerami, and R. Bucala, "Macrophage Migration Inhibitory Factor Is a Novel Mediator of Septic Shock," in *Proceedings of the 3rd International Congress on the Immune Consequences of Trauma, Shock, and Sepsis - Mechanisms and Therapeutic Approaches*, ed. E. Faist, A. Baue, and F. Shildberg (Scottsdale, AZ: Pabst Science Publishers, 1996), 394–96.
18. The Ninth MIF Symposium was held in Munich in October 2018. It seemed wholly appropriate that the immunologist John David gave the keynote speech at the Munich meeting, entitled "Half a Century of MIF Research," because John had been involved with research on the cytokine from the very beginning. John David was also an important element within Ken War-

ren's Great Neglected Diseases Network, and it was Ken who persuaded John "to explore the tanged fields of immunoparasitology."

19. Letter from Peter H. Raven (National Academy of Sciences) to Cerami, June 17, 1992 (Anthony Cerami personal papers).

20. Interview with Miki Rifkin, March 2018.

21. Interview with Anthony Cerami, October 2018.

22. P. Rosenfield, *A World of Giving: Carnegie Corporation of New York—A Century of International Philanthropy* (New York: Public Affairs, 2014), 1.

23. M. Jacoby, "Foundations' Founder yet to Donate $67-Million," *St Petersburg Times*, December 29, 2001.

24. Jacoby.

25. M. Bianchi, P. Ulrich, O. Bloom, et al., "An Inhibitor of Macrophage Arginine Transport and Nitric Oxide Production (CNI-1493) Prevents Acute Inflammation and Endotoxin Lethality," *Molecular Medicine* 1, no. 3 (1995): 254–66.

26. D. Gelles and G. Tett, "From behind Bars, Madoff Spins His Story," *The Financial Times*, April 8, 2011. Jeffry Picower, rather than Madoff, appeared to have been the largest beneficiary of the Madoff Ponzi scheme, and his estate settled the claims against it for $7.2 billion. His lawyers maintain he was unaware of the fraud. Jeffry Picower died on October 25, 2009, at his Palm Beach home—he suffered a heart attack while in the swimming pool, resulting in his drowning.

27. Interview with Charles Dinarello, February 2017.

28. C. Keating, *Kenneth Warren and the Great Neglected Diseases of Mankind Programme: The Transformation of Geographical Medicine in the US and Beyond* (Cham, Switzerland: Springer, 2017), 128.

29. Interview with Charles Dinarello, February 2017.

30. Interview with Barbara Sherry, May 2016.

11. TRANSLATION IN TRANSITION

Note to Epigraph: Sydenham quoting Hippocrates in G. Meynell, "John Locke and the Preface to Thomas Sydenham's Observationes Medicae," *Medical History* 50, no. 1 (2006): 105.

1. T. Kuhn, *The Structure of Scientific Revolutions* (Chicago: University of Chicago Press, 1962), 38.

2. I. Edwards, "How a Major Research Institute Got to Long Island," *New York Times*, September 1, 1991.

3. Interview with Anthony Cerami, December 2018.

4. Interview with Barbara Sherry, May 2016.

5. Interview with Loretta Itri, June 2019.

6. Interview with Pietro Ghezzi, March 2017.

7. Interview with Anthony Cerami, December 2018.

8. S. Lewis, *Arrowsmith* (New York: Signet Classics, 2008), 279.

9. At Rockefeller University, Mike Brines had written his thesis under the supervision of zoologist Donald Griffin. Griffin, in his book *Listening in the Dark*, published in 1958, described how bats seek and catch their insect prey in the dark via a process he described as "echolocation." Griffin was a brilliant and controversial scientist who pioneered the idea of animal consciousness. In the 1970s, Brines was studying how bees navigated their way from Rockefeller University to Central Park to find honey and then returned in the evening to his lab in Theobald Smith Hall, which was situated nine floors above Cerami's subterranean laboratory.

10. C. Cerami, H. Founds, I. Nicholl, et al., "Tobacco Smoke Is a Source of Toxic Reactive Glycation Products," *Proceedings of the National Academy of Sciences of the United States of America* 94, no. 25 (1997): 13915–20.

11. Interview with Mike Brines, June 2016.

12. Interview with Peter Ulrich, September 2018.

13. Interview with Mike Brines, June 2016.

14. Stuart O. Schweitzer in his scholarly work *Pharmaceutical Economics and Policy* (Oxford: Oxford University Press, 2007) describes the complex interrelationship between Amgen, the Kirin Brewery Co. of Japan, and Johnson & Johnson's Ortho Pharmaceutical Corporation. In 1985, the 50–50 joint venture between Amgen and Kirin allowed Johnson & Johnson to have worldwide manufacturing and marketing rights for genetically engineered erythropoietin, Epogen, Amgen's first product under development product sales. Kirin retained the rights to sell Epogen in Japan and China, and Ortho and Johnson & Johnson retained the rights to sell the product for some indications in the United States. Specifically, the marketing agreement granted Amgen the rights to sell Epogen to U.S. patients undergoing kidney dialysis, while Ortho retained the rights to sell Epogen in the United States for all other uses, including kidney patients not on dialysis treatment. Amgen sold Epogen in the United States for kidney patients, while Johnson & Johnson sold it under the trade name Procrit to treat patients experiencing renal insufficiency, patients with anemia caused by cancer treatment, surgery patients, and patients with AIDS. In 2000, Epogen had worldwide sales of about $4 billion.

15. A. Cerami, "A Surprising Journey in Translational Medicine," *Molecular Medicine* 20 (2014): S3.

16. Erythropoietin is secreted by the kidney and stimulates red blood cell production in the bone marrow. Recombinant human erythropoietin (rhEPO) is produced by recombinant DNA technology.

17. Interview with Loretta Itri, June 2019.

18. S. Schweitzer, *Pharmaceutical Economics and Policy* (New York: Oxford University Press, 2007), 58.

19. Interview with Loretta Itri, June 2019.

20. Interview with Loretta Itri, June 2019.

21. Interview with Loretta Itri, June 2019.

22. M. Brines, "Discovery of a Master Regulator of Injury and Healing: Tipping the Outcome from Damage toward Repair," *Molecular Medicine* 20 (2014): S11.

23. A. Cerami, "A Forty-Year Odyssey in the Sea of Translational Medicine," *Proceedings of the American Philosophical Society* 158, no. 4 (December 2014): 407.

24. Brines, "Discovery of a Master Regulator," S11.

25. M. Brines, P. Ghezzi, S. Keenan, et al., "Erythropoietin Crosses the Blood-Brain Barrier to Protect against Experimental Brain Injury," *Proceedings of the National Academy of Sciences of the United States of America* 97, no. 19 (2000): 10526–31.

26. Interview with Mike Brines, June 2016.

27. S. Masuda, M. Okano, K. Yamagishi, M. Nagao, M. Ueda, and R. Sasaki, "A Novel Site of Erythropoietin Production: Oxygen-Dependent Production in Cultured Rat Astrocytes," *Journal of Biological Chemistry* 269, no. 30 (1994): 19488–93.

28. Brines, "Discovery of a Master Regulator," S11.

29. Interview with Anthony Cerami, December 2018.

30. Interview with Siamon Gordon, January 2016.

31. S. Wolpe, G. Davatelis, B. Sherry, et al., "Macrophages Secrete a Novel Heparin-Binding Protein with Inflammatory and Neutrophil Chemokinetic Properties," *Journal of Experimental Medicine* 167, no. 2 (1988): 570–81.

32. Serendipity, or good luck, can play an essential part in the career of a scientist. Just such an event happened to Sir Peter Ratcliffe FRS in 1990 when his first ever paper on the subject of erythropoietin was published in the *JEM*. At the time, Tony Cerami was on the board of the journal and his remit was to broaden the *JEM*'s subject matter. The paper, which related to the production of EPO by isolated perfused kidneys, helped Ratcliffe to secure a senior fellowship from the Wellcome Trust. Ratcliffe is one of the world's leading physician-scientists, and in

2016, he won the Lasker Prize for discovering the mechanisms by which cells sense and signal hypoxia (low oxygen levels). His lab defined the oxygen sensing and signaling pathways that link the essential transcription factor, hypoxia-inducible factors (HIFs), to the available oxygen. Ratcliffe's work on the gene expression of erythropoietin opened up the new field of hypoxia. Hypoxia is an important component of many human diseases, including cancer, heart disease, stroke, vascular disease, and anemia. The importance of this work was fully recognized in October 2019 when Ratcliffe shared the Nobel Prize in Physiology or Medicine with William Kaelin Jr. at the Dana-Farber Cancer Institute and Harvard University, as well as Gregg Semenza at Johns Hopkins University, for their work describing how cells sense falling oxygen levels and respond by making new blood cells and vessels.

33. A. Cerami, "The Value of Failure: The Discovery of TNF and Its Natural Inhibitor Erythropoietin," *Journal of Internal Medicine* 269, no. 1 (2011): 8–15. Inflammation with innate immune system activation has been shown to directly activate HIF-1: see, for example, the review by V. Nizet and R. Johnson, "Interdependence of Hypoxic and Innate Immune Responses," *Nature Reviews Immunology* 9, no. 9 (2009): 609–17.

34. D. Weatherall, *Science and the Quiet Art: Medical Research and Patient Care* (Oxford: Oxford University Press, 1995), 181.

35. Interview with Loretta Itri, June 2019.

36. Interview with Anthony Cerami, June 2018.

37. Interview with Anthony Cerami, June 2018.

38. The British epidemiologist Sir Richard Peto FRS, in his study of mortality from noncommunicable diseases (NCDs), defines middle age as between thirty-five and sixty-nine.

39. Interview with Keith McAdam, August 2014.

40. Interview with Mike Brines, June 2016.

41. Interview with Anthony Cerami, June 2018.

42. Interview with Mike Brines, June 2016.

43. Interview with Loretta Itri, June 2019.

44. Interview with Anthony Cerami, June 2018.

45. Interview with Tom Coleman, May 2016.

46. On Tuesday, September 11, 2018, the Department of Justice U.S. Attorney's Office of the District of Massachusetts made this announcement: "The CEO of a microcap company that claimed to own valuable patented drug delivery technology was sentenced today in federal court in Boston in connection with a scheme to manipulate the market for his company's publicly traded stock. Learned Jeremiah Hand, 59, of Durham, N.C., was sentenced by U.S. District Court Chief Judge Patti B. Saris to nine months in prison and one year of supervised release, with restitution to be determined at a later date. In August 2016, Hand pleaded guilty to conspiracy to commit securities fraud. In May 2018, his brother, Jehu Hand, 61, was convicted by a federal jury of conspiracy, securities fraud and wire fraud, and he is scheduled to be sentenced on Oct. 25, 2018. Their other brother, Adam Hand, 53, of Newport Beach, Calif., was sentenced to 30 months in prison and three years of supervised release after pleading guilty to one count of conspiracy to commit securities fraud. The Hand brothers conspired in a pump-and-dump scheme to manipulate the market for the stock of Crown Marketing, a microcap or 'penny stock' company that claimed to own valuable patented drug delivery technology. Specifically, Learned Hand and his brothers engaged in a scheme to conceal their control over the majority of Crown's free-trading stock so that they could 'pump' up the company's share price and then secretly 'dump' their shares into the market."

47. Interview with Tom Coleman, May 2016.

48. Interview with Anthony Cerami, May 2016.

49. H. Corwin, H. Gettinger, T. Fabian, et al., "Efficacy and Safety of Epoetin Alfa in Critically Ill Patients," *New England Journal of Medicine* 357, no. 10 (2007): 965–76.

50. Cerami, "Forty-Year Odyssey," 406.

51. P. Whoriskey, "Anemia Drug Made Billions, but at What Cost?" *Washington Post*, July 19, 2012.

52. Interview with Anthony Cerami, June 2018.

53. M. Brines, G. Grasso, F. Fiordaliso, et al., "Erythropoietin Mediates Tissue Protection through an Erythropoietin and Common Beta-Subunit Heteroreceptor," *Proceedings of the National Academy of Sciences of the United States of America* 101, no. 41 (2004): 14907–12.

54. S. Erbayraktar, G. Grasso, A. Stacteria, et al., "Asialoerythropoietin Is a Non-Erythropoietin Cytokine with Broad Neuroprotective Activity *In Vivo*," *Proceedings of the National Academy of Sciences of the United States of America* 100, no. 11 (2003): 6741–46.

55. G. Ferry, "Sydney Brenner Obituary," *The Guardian*, April 5, 2018.

56. M. Leist, P. Ghezzi, G. Grasso, et al., "Derivatives of Erythropoietin That Are Tissue Protective but Not Erythropoietic," *Science* 305, no. 5681 (2004): 239–42.

57. Thomas Coleman is the son of Douglas Coleman, a colleague of Cerami's in the late 1960s at the Jackson Laboratory. Tom and Carla played together as children in Acadia National Park, Bar Harbor, Maine.

58. Interview with Tom Coleman, May 2016.

59. T. Coleman, C. Westenfelder, F. Togel, et al., "Cytoprotective Doses of Erythropoietin or Carbamylated Erythropoietin Have Markedly Different Procoagulant and Vasoactive Activities," *Proceedings of the National Academy of Sciences of the United States of America* 103, no. 15 (2006): 5965–70.

60. Interview with Loretta Itri, June 2019.

61. Interview with Tom Coleman, May 2016.

62. The KSWI could not get access to EPO itself because of the patent situation whereby Amgen and J&J held the commercial rights in both the United States and Europe.

63. Interview with Mike Brines, June 2016.

64. Shire was acquired by Japan's biggest pharmaceutical company Takeda for £46 billion in 2018.

65. Interview with Mike Brines, June 2016.

66. When the Shire agreement was terminated, Warren Pharma could not find another partner to fund the very expensive development program requiring biological products (proteins). As Mike Brines has written, "Given the lack of success getting a partner for Warren Pharma, we thought that the best chance of success for Warren Pharma shareholders would be [the] success of its subsidiary Araim Pharma. So, while efforts continued to find a way forward for Warren Pharma, the Araim Pharma development programme was vigorously pursued."

67. M. Brines, N. Patel, P. Villa, et al., "Nonerythropoietic, Tissue-Protective Peptides Derived from the Tertiary Structure of Erythropoietin," *Proceedings of the National Academy of Sciences of the United States of America* 105, no. 31 (2008): 19025–30.

12. ANTI-TNF THERAPY

1. L. Marks, "The Birth Pangs of Monoclonal Antibody Therapeutics: The Failure and Legacy of Centoxin," *mAbs* 4, no. 3 (2012): 403–12.

2. There are principally three ways in which antibodies achieve their effectiveness as therapeutics. First, it is to bind and block the activity of whatever the target is, another is to kill where it is attached by recruiting a variety of cells in the immune system, and a third way is by a very important feature of antibodies—their very long half-life. Whereas a small molecule will be filtered out of the body by the kidneys very quickly, a large molecule such as an antibody can stay around in the circulation for several weeks.

3. Interview with Greg Winter, October 2014.

4. J. Vilcek, "First Demonstration of the Role of TNF in the Pathogenesis of Disease," *Journal of Immunology* 181, no. 1 (2008): 5–6.

5. Interview with Jan Vilcek, April 2015. The original paper may be found in B. Beutler, I. Milsark, and A. Cerami, "Passive Immunization against Cachectin/Tumor Necrosis Factor Protects Mice from Lethal Effect of Endotoxin," *Science* 229, no. 4716 (1985): 869–71.

6. Interview with Jan Vilcek, April 2015.

7. D. Knight, H. Trinh, J. Le, et al., "Construction and Initial Characterization of a Mouse-Human Chimeric Anti-TNF Antibody," *Molecular Immunology* 30, no. 16 (1993): 1443–53.

8. Interview with Jan Vilcek, April 2015.

9. Interview with Jim Woody, September 2013.

10. Interview with Jan Vilcek, April 2015.

11. D. Davis, *The Beautiful Cure: Harnessing Your Body's Natural Defences* (London: The Bodley Head, 2018), 83.

12. Interview with Gus Nossal, September 2013.

13. Interview with Gus Nossal, September 2013.

14. Davis, *The Beautiful Cure*, 95.

15. Interview with Jim Woody, September 2013.

16. F. Brennan, D. Chantry, A. Jackson, R. Maini, and M. Feldmann, "Inhibitory Effect of TNF Alpha Antibodies on Synovial Cell Interleukin-1 Production in Rheumatoid Arthritis," *Lancet* 2, no. 8657 (1989): 244–47.

17. Interview with Jim Woody, September 2013.

18. M. Feldmann, "Development of Anti-TNF Therapy for Rheumatoid Arthritis," *Nature Reviews Immunology* 2, no. 5 (2002): 364–71.

19. NIH-funded trials have a success rate of approximately one in ten.

20. Interview with Jim Woody, September 2013.

21. C. Keating, *Great Medical Discoveries: An Oxford Story* (Oxford: The Bodleian Library, 2013), 49.

22. Interview with Ravinder Maini, September 2013.

23. Interview with Jim Woody, September 2013.

24. Interview with Jan Vilcek, April 2015.

25. Interview with Ravinder Maini, September 2013.

26. Interview with Jim Woody, September 2013.

27. Davis, *The Beautiful Cure*.

28. M. Elliott, R. Maini, M. Feldmann, et al., "Repeated Therapy with Monoclonal Antibody to Tumor Necrosis Factor Alpha (cA2) in Patients with Rheumatoid Arthritis," *Lancet* 344, no. 8930 (1994): 1125–27.

29. M. Elliott, R. Maini, M. Feldmann, et al., "Randomised Double-Blind Comparison of Chimeric Monoclonal Antibody to Tumor Necrosis Factor Alpha (cA2) versus Placebo in Rheumatoid Arthritis," *Lancet* 344, no. 8930 (1994): 1105–10.

30. R. Maini, F. Breedveld, J. Kalden, et al., "Therapeutic Efficacy of Multiple Intravenous Infusions of Anti-Tumor Necrosis Factor Alpha Monoclonal Antibody Combined with Low-Dose Weekly Methotrexate in Rheumatoid Arthritis," *Arthritis and Rheumatism* 41, no. 9 (1998): 1552–63.

31. Interview with Ravinder Maini, September 2013.

32. Interview with David Isenberg, July 2014.

33. The first of the biologic drugs that blocked TNF was Enbrel (etanercept), Remicade (infliximab), and Humira (adalimumab), introduced between 1998 and 2002.

34. Feldmann, "Development of Anti-TNF Therapy," 364–71.

35. Interview with Ferdinand Breedveld, May 2016.

36. Interview with Kevin Tracey, August 2017.

37. Interview with Jan Vilcek, April 2015.

13. TAKING ON BIG PHARMA

1. S. Prideaux, *I Am Dynamite! The Life of Friedrich Nietzsche* (London: Faber & Faber, 2018), 389.

2. Interview with Tom Coleman, May 2016.

3. Civ. Action No. 2: 04-cv 168 (TJV) (Anthony Cerami personal papers).

4. Interview with Charles Dinarello, February 2017.

5. Interview with Charles Dinarello, February 2017.

6. Email from Lee Nadler to Conrad Keating, August 2019.

7. Interview with Charles Dinarello, February 2017.

8. Interview with Charles Dinarello, February 2017.

9. E. Joshua Rosenkranz, counsel for Dr. Anthony Cerami 09-2921-cv p 5. In United States Court of Appeals for the Second Circuit (December 4, 2009) (Anthony Cerami personal papers).

10. Interview with Masanobu Kawakami, August 2017.

11. Court transcript (Anthony Cerami personal papers).

12. Cerami and Kawakami's original patent (U.S. 6419927 B1) was filed on September 8, 1981, and entitled "Method for Reducing Adverse Effects of a Human 70KDA Mediator Which Results from Endotoxin Stimulation of Macrophages." The abstract read, "Provided are therapeutic uses of antibodies capable of neutralizing the adverse effects in humans of the about 70kDa mediator produced upon invasive stimulation of macrophages by, e.g. contact with endotoxin."

13. In a letter from Edward E. Penhoet to Cerami dated February 4, 1985, Penhoet wrote, "During the research and development phases, Chiron expects to compensate you as a consultant at a minimum of $12,000 per year, and to allow you to participate in a stock option program for consultants. . . . We are very excited about this project and with the prospect of collaborating with you. I'm hopeful we'll be able to meet with Mr Griesar [a Rockefeller lawyer] in the very near future to finalize an agreement and that we'll be able to begin the science before the end of the month."

14. Letter from Edward E. Penhoet to Cerami, August 16, 1985 (Anthony Cerami personal papers).

15. Interview with Jan Vilcek, April 2015.

16. M. Elliott, R. Maini, M. Feldmann, et al., "Randomised Double-Blind Comparison of Chimeric Monoclonal Antibody to Tumor Necrosis Factor Alpha (cA2) versus Placebo in Rheumatoid Arthritis," *Lancet* 344, no. 8930 (1994): 1105–10.

17. Interview with Ferdinand Breedveld, May 2016.

18. E. Joshua Rosenkranz, counsel for Dr. Anthony Cerami 09-2921-cv p 2. In United States Court of Appeals for the Second Circuit (December 4, 2009) (Anthony Cerami personal papers).

19. 09-2921-cv. In United States Court of Appeals for the Second Circuit. Brief of Plaintiff-Appellee, 1 (Anthony Cerami personal papers).

20. 09-2921-cv. In United States Court of Appeals for the Second Circuit. Brief of Plaintiff-Appellee, 1 (Anthony Cerami personal papers).

21. Interview with Sharon Stern, July 2019.

22. Interview with Mike Brines, July 2019.

23. 09-2921-cv. In United States Court of Appeals for the Second Circuit. Brief of Plaintiff-Appellee, 55 (Anthony Cerami personal papers).

24. 09-2921-cv. In United States Court of Appeals for the Second Circuit. Brief of Plaintiff-Appellee, 55 (Anthony Cerami personal papers).

25. Interview with Sharon Stern, July 2019.

26. Interview with Ann Dunne, August 2019.

27. 09-2921-cv. Reply brief of Defendant—Appellant Novartis Vaccines and Diagnostics, Inc. Evan R. Chesler. Cravath, Swaine and Moore LLP (February 1, 2010), 4 (Anthony Cerami personal papers).

28. Interview with Sharon Stern, July 2019.

29. *The American Lawyer*, January 2012.

30. Interview with Sharon Stern, July 2019.

31. C. Bray, "Biochemist Sues Novartis, Unit over Royalty Payments," *Market Watch*, June 14, 2007.

32. 09-2921-cv. Reply brief of Defendant—Appellant Novartis Vaccines and Diagnostics, Inc. Evan R. Chesler. Cravath, Swaine and Moore LLP (February 1, 2010), 15 (Anthony Cerami personal papers).

33. The case had a personal resonance for Rosenkranz. His own father was a renowned cancer research scientist who had made numerous discoveries but had been reluctant to capitalize on them. However, on the one occasion that he launched a joint venture to commercialize a procedure that he had developed, through a series of financial and legal maneuvers, the investors collected all of the proceeds and his father was left with nothing. Rozenkranz felt that Novartis had taken a highly valuable discovery and made a lot of money from it but thought it could marginalize Cerami's contribution. For his part, Cerami knew exactly what he had contributed scientifically and was not embarrassed about fighting for it. Novartis had probably not expected Cerami to go the whole distance and take them on in a court of law. But Cerami had an abiding faith in the justice system to yield the right result. He already had a jury verdict, and he remained steadfast in his belief that his position would ultimately be vindicated. At the appeal, Rosenkranz had an unshakable belief that "Tony was right, the jury verdict was just and the trial was fair."

34. The name Araim was chosen because it was a play on "our aim"—however, Tom Coleman thought that Cerami should not have opted for an onomatopoeic nomenclature but chosen instead "ANCER" as it was an immensely appropriate name for a biological startup while having the added attraction of incorporating the founder's name.

35. Carla Cerami became a successful tropical disease researcher focusing on the innate immune response to malaria infection and injury. She worked both at the MRC Unit Gambia (Sir Brian Greenwood, a former director of the unit and a champion of medical education and development in Africa, was on Carla's interview panel), which was established in 1947, and at the University of North Carolina, Chapel Hill with Steve Meshnick.

36. Interview with Mike Brines, July 2019.

37. A. Sinclair, A. Coxon, I. McCaffery, et al., "Functional Erythropoietin Receptor Is Undetectable in Endothelial, Cardiac, Neuronal, and Renal Cells," *Blood* 115, no. 21 (2010): 4264–72.

38. Interview with Mike Brines, July 2019.

39. P. Ghezzi, M. Bernaudin, R. Bianchi, et al., "Erythropoietin: Not Just about Erythropoiesis," *Lancet* 375, no. 9732 (2010): 2142.

40. L. Siren, M. Fratelli, M. Brines, et al., "Erythropoietin Prevents Neuronal Apoptosis after Cerebral Ischemia and Metabolic Stress," *Proceedings of the National Academy of Sciences of the United States of America* 98, no. 7 (2001): 4044–49.

41. C. Ott, H. Martens, I. Hassouna, et al., "Widespread Expression of Erythropoietin Receptor in Brain and Its Induction by Injury," *Molecular Medicine* 21, no. 1 (2015): 803–15.

42. Herman Boerhaave (1668–1738) was a Dutch botanist, chemist, and an exponent of bedside teaching. He became known as "the father of physiology," and his influence was instrumental in establishing the fame of the school of medicine at the University of Leiden. He gave his name to *Boerhaave syndrome*, the rupture of the esophagus bought about by severe vomiting.

43. In August 2008, Cerami and Annie Dunne arrived in Leiden carrying two suitcases each. For the first eighteen months, Cerami was traveling back and forth to the United States twice a month to visit his daughter Angelina. Meanwhile, Annie's daughter Sage (Sage Dunne-Cerami) settled into secondary school in Leiden, where she quickly learned Dutch and how to ride a bike safely through the congested canal-lined streets of the city.

44. Interview with Albert Dahan, May 2016.

45. A. Dahan, M. Brines, M. Niesters, A. Cerami, and M. van Velzen, "Targeting the Innate Repair Receptor to Treat Neuropathy," *Pain Reports* 1, no. 1 (2016): e566.

46. A. Dahan, A. Dunne, M. Swartjes, et al., "ARA 290 Improves Symptoms in Patients with Sarcoidosis-Associated Small Nerve Fibre Loss and Increases Corneal Nerve Fibre Density," *Molecular Medicine* 19, no. 1 (2013): 334–45.

47. Interview with Albert Dahan, May 2016.

48. M. Brines and A. Cerami, "The Receptor That Tames the Innate Immune Response," *Molecular Medicine* 18, no. 1 (2012): 486–96.

49. Interview with Chris Thiemermann, September 2016.

50. M. Coldewey, S. Khan, A. Kapoor, et al., "Erythropoietin Attenuates Acute Kidney Dysfunction in Murine Experimental Sepsis by Activation of the b-Common Receptor," *Kidney International* 84, no. 3 (2013): 482–90; M. Collino, C. Thiemermann, A. Cerami, and M. Brines, "Flipping the Molecular Switch for Innate Protection and Repair of Tissues: Long-lasting Effects of a Non-Erythropoietic Small Peptide Engineered from Erythropoietin," *Pharmacology & Therapeutics* 151 (2015): 32–40.

51. Ostenson used the Japanese rat Goto-Kakizaki (GK) in his experiments.

52. M. Watanabe, T. Lundgren, Y. Saito, et al., "A Nonhematopoietic Erythropoietin Analogue, ARA 290, Inhibits Macrophage Activation and Prevents Damage to Transplanted Islets," *Transplantation* 100, no. 3 (2016): 554–62.

53. Interview with Alan Fairlamb, May 2016.

54. Interview with Mike Brines, July 2019.

55. Interview with Chris Thiemermann, September 2016.

56. Interview with Mike Brines, July 2019.

57. L. Heij, M. Niesters, M. Swartjes, et al., "Safety and Efficacy of ARA 290 in Sarcoidosis Patients with Symptoms of Small Fiber Neuropathy: A Randomized, Double-Blind Pilot Study," *Molecular Medicine* 18, no. 1 (2012): 1430–36.

58. Interview with Alan Fairlamb, May 2016.

59. Interview with Chas Bountra, August 2018.

60. P. de Kruif, *Microbe Hunters* (New York: Blue Ribbon Books, 1926), 358.

61. B. Gilmer, "Is It Still Possible to Be a Triple-Threat in Modern Medicine?" *Op-Med*, October 8, 2018.

62. The immunobiologist John David, a friend and colleague of Cerami from the GND era, referred to the triple threat as the *three-legged stool* but that in reality, "you can't be wonderful at all three, and remember to compete for grants you have to excel at the laboratory bench. You can't do all three and survive."

63. H. Kuchler, "Counting the Cost of America's Soaring Drug Prices," *FT Weekend*, September 21–22, 2019, 16.

64. J. DiMasi, H. Grabowski, and R. Hansen, "Innovation in the Pharmaceutical Industry: New Estimates of R&D Costs," *Journal of Health Economics* 47 (2016): 20–33.

65. Speech by Detlev Bronk in support of Anthony Cerami's doctorate in philosophy (June 1967).

66. Interview with Kevin Tracey, August 2016.

67. Speech by Detlev Bronk in support of Anthony Cerami's doctorate in philosophy (June 1967).

68. Interview with David Weatherall, August 2018.

INDEX

Note: Page references in *italics* refer to photographs.

Abbott Laboratories, 144–45, 147, 150–51
academic course at RIMR, 27
Ackerman, Samuel, 91
adipocytes, 83
admission to RIMR, 22–24
affluence, 16–17, 101–2
Africa, 1–2, 76–79, 83, 95–96, 108–9
AGE (advanced glycosylation end products), 56–70, 127–28, 160–61
aging, 55, 56–70, 75–76
agriculture, child labor in, 11–12
Alexander, Barbara (Ehrenreich), 31–32; *Living with a Wild God*, 31
Alteon, 66–67, 68–69
Amadori product, 52, 58–59, 64–65
ambition: of Bronk for The Rockefeller University, 21–22; of Cerami in translational medicine, 36; in Cerami's character, 34–35; in creativity, 107–8; for KSWI, 127, 131–32, 133–34; at The Rockefeller University, 35, 110–11; of Warren, for a tropical disease laboratory network, 71–72
American Dream, 11
Amgen, 134–35, 137, 152–53, 184n14
aminoguanidine, 64–70
anemia, 40–41, 47–49, 78, 79–85, 128–29. *See also* sickle cell disease/anemia; trypanosomes/trypanosomiasis
animal husbandry, 15
animal models, 6, 18–19, 81–82, 94–95, 97, 98–99, 141, 154
Anthony Cerami and Ann Dunne Foundation for World Health, 157
antibodies, monoclonal: as anti-TNF therapy, 84–85, 94–97, 99, 138, 139, 141, 142–43; discovery of, in profound change, 173n57; in injectable biologic therapeutics, 2; in patent litigation, 145
anticancer therapies: in summer job at Pfizer, 18–19; TNF as, 88–89, 90–91, 93, 94
anticytokine therapy, 98
anti-inflammatories, 122, 131–32, 151–53, 154–56

anti-TNF therapy, 2, 84–85, 94–97, 99–100, 138–43, 144–52
apprentice system, 106–7
ARA 290, 151–52, 153–55
Araim Pharmaceuticals, 137, 151–52, 153–56, 189n34
arteriosclerosis, 64–65, 66–67
Arthritis Research UK, 142
arts: in emotional literacy, 104; in RIMR's interdisciplinary approach, 22
asialo-EPO, 135, 137. *See also* EPO (erythropoietin)
ATP (adenosine triphosphate), 58
autonomy, 110–11, 114–15
Axel, Richard, 66

Baker, O. E., 11–12
Baltimore, David, 109–15
Baltimore Case, The, 111–12
Banting Medal of the American Diabetes Association, 54–55
barriers, overcome, in life and education, 15–16
beer: and science at PIMR, 117–18; and sociability at The Rockefeller University, 103
Bell, John, 72–73
bench-to-bedside factors, 3–4, 6
Bernstein, Gerald, 53, 54–55
Beutler, Bruce, 86–88, 89–93, 94–95, 145
Beutler, Ernest, 86–87
Big Pharma. *See* pharmaceutical industry
biochemistry: in evolution of molecular biology, 28–29; of parasites, in research on trypanosomiasis, 74–75; PhD program in, 119–20
biologics/biologic industry, 2, 7, 136–37, 138–40, 144–52. *See also* EPO (erythropoietin)
biology, human: Cerami's creativity in knowledge of, 128; evolution of, 86; RIMR in understanding of, 26–27, 76; understanding of, 36–37, 43–44

ABOUT THE AUTHOR

CONRAD KEATING is the writer-in-residence and visiting professor at the School of Medicine, Trinity College Dublin. Keating had previously been the writer-in-residence at the Wellcome Unit for the History of Medicine at the University of Oxford. His most recent publication is the widely acclaimed medical biography *Kenneth Warren and the Great Neglected Diseases of Mankind Program: The Transformation of Geographical Medicine in the US and Beyond* (2017). In 2013, Keating curated the exhibition "800 Years of Oxford Innovation: Great Medical Discoveries" for the Bodleian Library and wrote the accompanying book *Great Medical Discoveries: An Oxford Story* (2013). Keating's other major work in the history of medicine is *Smoking Kills: The Revolutionary Life of Richard Doll* (2009). Keating also has an Art of Medicine essay series on the history of randomized controlled trials in *The Lancet*; in April 2020, his article "A History of the RTS,S Malaria Vaccine" was published as the third essay in this ten-part series.

ABOUT THE AUTHOR

CONRAD KEATING is the writer-in-residence and visiting professor in the Sir William Dunn School of Medicine...